VITAMIX BLENDER COOKBOOK:

Blend Your Way to Culinary Excellence:
A Comprehensive Vitamix Cookbook.

Dr. Vera J. Reynolds

Copyright

This book is a work of non-fiction. The information, opinions, and advice presented in this book are based on the author's research and personal experience. The author and publisher make no representation or warranties with respect to the accuracy or completeness of the contents of this book and specifically disclaim any implied warranties of merchantability or fitness for a particular purpose.

The information contained in this book is provided on an "as is" basis and is intended to be used for general informational purposes only. The views and opinions expressed in this book are those of the author and do not necessarily reflect the official policy or position of any agency, organization, employer, or company.

Contents

INTRODUCTION

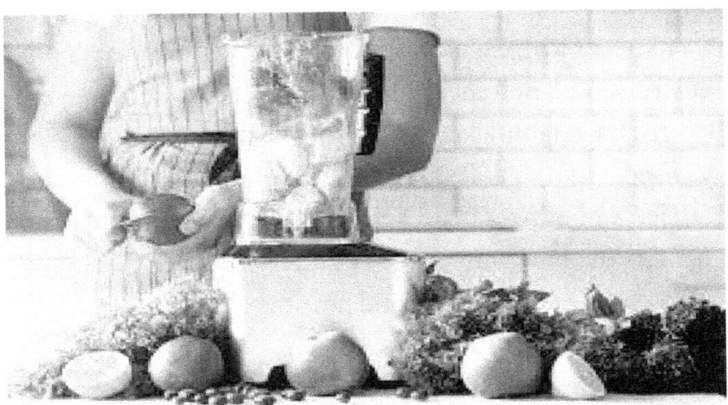

In the contemporary kitchen, where culinary creativity meets convenience, the Vitamix Blender is a vital cornerstone, ready to turn materials into culinary marvels. For those who aspire to blend, create, and enrich their gourmet experience, the Vitamix Blender is a genuine ally, giving a field of culinary possibilities limited only by one's imagination. This powerful and adaptable kitchen gadget transcends its position as a basic blender, emerging as a culinary instrument that allows amateur cooks and professional chefs alike to make a variety of concoctions that span the range from healthful breakfasts to indulgent desserts.

At its foundation, the Vitamix Blender is characterized by its remarkable performance and unrivalled accuracy. Engineered with cutting-edge technology, the core of the Vitamix is a high-powered engine that effortlessly pulverizes even the hardest of materials, resulting in smooth textures and consistent blends that set the bar for culinary perfection. From fibrous veggies to frozen fruits, Vitamix's blades seamlessly turn items into velvety purees, smooth soups, creamy dips, and more.

Beyond its technical excellence, the Vitamix Blender is also admired for its adaptability. Its flexibility transcends beyond culinary genres, enabling various dishes that appeal to different dietary needs and palates. Whether you want to produce nutrient-rich smoothies, vivid acai bowls, substantial soups, or even handmade nut butter, the Vitamix Blender rises with uncompromising performance and accuracy.

Yet, the actual magic of the Vitamix Blender rests not only in its mechanics but also in the culinary experiences it enables. From the delightful hum of the motor to the slow metamorphosis of ingredients, blending with a Vitamix becomes an art form, allowing the users to design harmonious combinations of tastes and textures that excite the senses. It is simplicity and easy controls allow beginners and seasoned chefs to go on culinary journeys, experimenting with ingredients and methods to produce meals that delight and inspire.

As you delve farther into the world of the Vitamix Blender, you'll find some recipes that celebrate its potential. From the refreshing embrace of morning smoothies to the warming comfort of blended soups, the Vitamix lifts the ordinary to the exceptional, bringing forth foods that feed the body and please the palette. The chapters ahead will walk you through an examination of this incredible appliance's potential, enabling you to uncover tastes, textures, and combinations that may have previously seemed out of reach.

As you immerse yourself in the world of the Vitamix Blender, prepare to go on a culinary adventure that surpasses conventional bounds. Each recipe encourages you to connect with your Vitamix as a creative collaborator, from healthy to decadent, from simple to complicated. This tool allows you to produce culinary experiences that convey your unique narrative. So, let the blending begin, and may your culinary undertakings be defined by the vibrancy, originality, and delight that the Vitamix Blender provides to your kitchen.

CHAPTER ONE

Understanding Blender Components

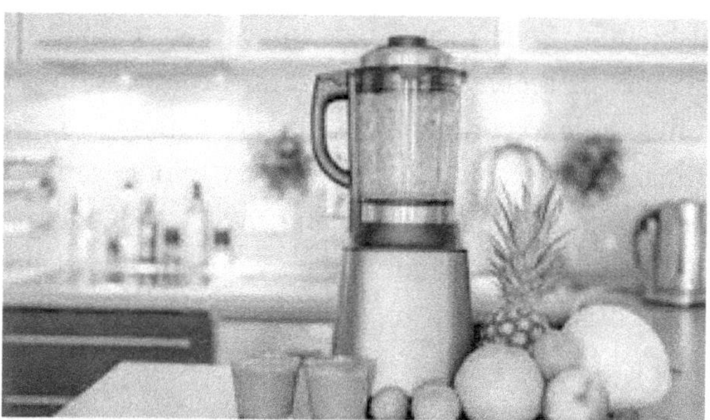

Blenders are multipurpose kitchen tools that make cooking and meal preparation more efficient. To properly harness the power of a Vitamix blender, it's essential to understand the numerous components that make up this equipment. Each member performs a particular function in the blending process, adding to the quality and consistency of your culinary creations. Let's look into the significant parts of your Vitamix blender:

1. **Motor Base and Power Ratings:** The motor base is the basis of the blender, containing the strong motor that powers the blades. Vitamix blenders are noted for their high-powered engines, measured in watts. The more the wattage, the more capable the blender is of handling difficult items like ice, frozen fruits, and nuts.

2. **Blender Jar & Materials:** The blender jar, commonly built from sturdy materials like BPA-free Tritan plastic

or tempered glass, retains the contents during mixing. Vitamix blender jars are made to endure the high-speed blending process and the impact of solid components.

3. **Blades and Cutting Mechanism:** The edges are at the core of the mixing process. Vitamix blenders generally include stainless steel blades that handle wet and dry components. These blades generate a vortex that draws materials toward the center for thorough mixing.

4. **Control Panel and Settings:** Vitamix blenders come with a control panel offering several settings that govern the speed and length of blending. Some versions provide pre-programmed settings for specialized jobs, including smoothies, soups, and more. Manual speed control enables you to modify the mixing speed as desired.

5. **Lid and Tamper Functions:** The blender lid serves a dual purpose: it stops components from splattering during blending and features a detachable lid plug that lets you add ingredients while mixing. The tamper, a unique feature of Vitamix blenders, helps move materials about the jar, guaranteeing smooth blending, even with dense combinations.

Understanding how each component contributes to the blending process will allow you to produce a broad assortment of recipes with your Vitamix blender. Whether you're cooking silky smoothies, creamy soups, or nut butter, understanding how to use these components can improve your culinary experience.

Proper maintenance and treatment of these components are equally crucial. Regularly cleaning the jar, lid, blades, and base ensures that your blender stays in outstanding condition, consistently performing for years to come. By familiarizing yourself with the components and understanding their functions, you'll be well-equipped to explore the fantastic world of blending possibilities that your Vitamix blender provides.

Essential Blender Techniques

Blending is an art that goes beyond just blending components. Mastering basic blender methods may lift your culinary creations to new heights. With a Vitamix blender as your tool, you have the power to produce silky textures, robust flavours, and stunning presentations. Let's discuss some essential approaches that can help you get the most out of your blending experience:

1. **Blending vs. Pulse Function:** Understanding when to use the continuous blending mode and when to employ the pulse function is critical. Continuous blending is excellent for making silky purees, while the pulse function enables you to generate coarse textures or avoid over-blending.

2. **Gradual Ingredient Addition:** For best mixing, add components gradually. Start with liquids or soft parts in the bottom of the jar to simplify the blending process. As you add additional ingredients, the vortex

generated by the blades will attract everything into the center for complete mixing.

3. **Achieving Smooth Textures:** To produce silky smooth textures, mix at high speed for an acceptable length. This approach works great for generating creamy soups, sauces, and smoothies without any apparent lumps.

4. **Creating Texture Variations:** If you're trying for a chunkier texture, mix at a lower speed for shorter intervals. This approach is ideal for salsas, dips, and dishes where you want unique ingredient textures.

5. **Blending Hot substances Safely:** Exercise care to minimize pressure development when blending hot liquids or substances. Leave the lid stopper slightly open to enable steam to escape, or agree at a lower speed to avoid the chance of splattering.

6. **Emulsification and Homogenization:** The high-speed blending action of your Vitamix can emulsify oil and liquids, making creamy dressings and sauces. Start by mixing the liquid components and gently trickle in the oil while the mixer runs to obtain a steady emulsion.

Learning five essential blender methods allows you to make various recipes that appeal to varied tastes and textures. Experiment with multiple ingredient combinations, blending durations, and speeds to produce the desired results. Your

Vitamix blender is a powerful instrument that may help you reach culinary perfection with every blend.

Remember that practice makes perfect. As you become more comfortable with these methods, you'll develop the confidence to modify them to your culinary tastes and create meals that astound and please.

Care & Maintenance of Your Vitamix

Proper care and maintenance are necessary to maintain your Vitamix blender functioning at its best and prolonging its lifetime. By following these maintenance requirements, you'll ensure consistent blending results and enjoy your blender's capabilities for years.

1. **Regular Cleaning:**
   - After each use, dismantle your blender, wash the jar lid, and tamper with warm soapy water.
   - Rinse well to eliminate any residue.
   - Avoid soaking the motor base in water; wipe it off with a wet towel.
2. **Thorough Cleaning:** Periodically, thoroughly clean the blender jar with warm water and a few drops of dish soap. Run the blender quickly for 30-60 seconds, then rinse well. This helps clean the blades, container, and seals properly.

3. **Removing Tough Residue:** For harsh residue, use warm water and baking soda to assist in dislodging deposits.

Alternatively, use a combination of water and vinegar for mineral buildup. Follow up with a thorough rinse.

4. **Storing the Blender:** When not in use, keep the blender with the lid slightly ajar to promote air circulation and avoid smells. Store the jar and lid separately to avoid trapping moisture.

5. **Maintaining Blades and Seals:** Check the blades for symptoms of dullness or damage. If required, Vitamix sells new blade assemblies. Regularly examine the seals for wear and tear, and replace them if they become cracked or broken to avoid leaks.

6. **Avoid overflowing:** Follow the suggested ingredient amounts to avoid drowning the jar. Overloading might strain the motor and compromise mixing efficiency.

7. **Blending Hot Ingredients:** When blending hot liquids, start at a low speed and gradually raise it to minimize pressure building. Remove the lid stopper or leave it slightly open to release steam.

8. **Troubleshooting:** Check the user manual or Vitamix customer care for advice if your blender develops troubles. Only dismantle the motor base if advised by support staff.

9. **Warranty Information:** Familiarize yourself with your blender's warranty terms. Vitamix blenders frequently

come with extended warranties that cover multiple components.

10. **Upkeep of Motor Base:** Keep the motor base dry and prevent exposure to moisture. If any liquid falls onto the ground, unplug the blender and wipe it dry immediately.

By sticking to these care and maintenance methods, you'll guarantee that your Vitamix blender stays in great shape and continues to offer consistent blending results. A well-maintained blender assures superior performance and increases your whole cooking and mixing experience.

CHAPTER TWO

Breakfast Blends

Tropical Sunrise Smoothie:

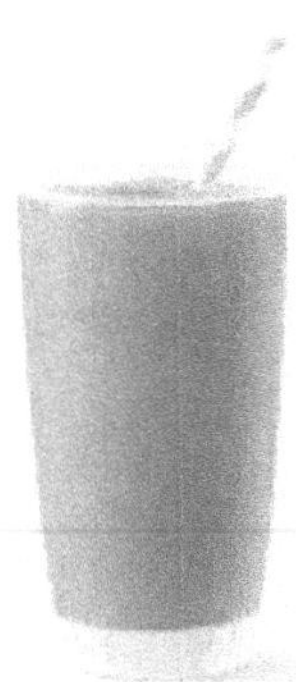

Start your day with a rush of tropical tastes and refreshing bliss. This Tropical Sunrise Smoothie mixes the lively sweetness of pineapple and mango with the smoothness of banana and Greek yogurt, all heightened by the tangy brightness of orange juice. It's like a drink of sunlight to boost your morning!

Ingredients:

- 1 cup chopped pineapple (fresh or frozen)
- ½ cup chopped mango (fresh or frozen)
- 1 ripe banana
- ½ cup Greek yogurt
- ½ cup orange juice

- Ice cubes (optional)

Instructions:

Prepare the Ingredients:

- If using fresh pineapple and mango, wash, peel, and cube them.
- Peel the ripe banana and split it into bits.
- Measure out the Greek yogurt and orange juice.

Blend It Up:

- Add the chopped pineapple, mango, banana, Greek yogurt, and orange juice to your Vitamix mixer.

Optional: Add Ice:

- Add a handful of ice cubes to the blender if you like a colder and thicker texture.

Blend Until Smooth:

- Start mixing on low speed and gradually raise to high.
- Blend until all the ingredients are well integrated, and the result is smooth and creamy.

Taste and Adjust:

- If desired, give the smoothie a taste and modify the sweetness or tanginess by adding more banana or orange juice.

Serve and Enjoy:

- Pour the Tropical Sunrise Smoothie into glasses.
- Optionally, you may garnish with a piece of pineapple or a sprinkling of shredded coconut.

- Try freezing the banana and adding frozen pineapple and mango pieces to make it even more refreshing.

This Tropical Sunrise Smoothie is tasty and filled with vitamins, fibre, and natural energy. It's a great way to spice up your morning ritual and give yourself a healthy boost to start the day.

Berry Burst Oat Smoothie

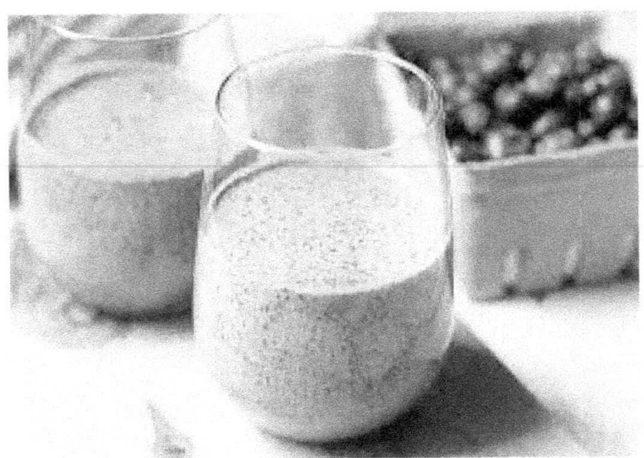

Indulge in the fantastic mixture of rich mixed berries and nourishing rolled oats with this Berry Burst Oat Smoothie. Packed with antioxidants, fibre, and natural sweetness, this smoothie is tasty and fulfilling, making it an excellent option for a healthy breakfast or a refreshing snack.

Ingredients:

- 1 cup mixed berries (strawberries, blueberries, raspberries, etc.; fresh or frozen)
- ½ cup rolled oats

- 1 cup almond milk (or milk of your choice)
- One tablespoon almond butter (or nut butter of your choice)
- One tablespoon of honey or maple syrup (optional for extra sweetness)
- Ice cubes (optional)

Instructions:

Prepare the Ingredients:

- If using fresh berries, wash and remove any stems. If using frozen berries, there's no need to defrost them.
- Measure out the rolled oats, almond milk, almond butter, and sweetener (if using).

Blend the Base:

- Add the mixed berries, rolled oats, almond milk, almond butter, and sweetener (if using) to your Vitamix blender.

Optional: Add Ice:

- Add a few ice cubes to the blender if you like a colder and thicker texture.

Blend Until Smooth:

- Start mixing on low speed and gradually raise to high.
- Blend until the sauce is smooth and all the components are properly blended.

Taste and Adjust:

- Give the smoothie a taste and adjust the sweetness or thickness by adding additional honey, almond milk, or oats as desired.

- Pour the Berry Burst Oat Smoothie into glasses.
- Optionally, top with fresh berries or a sprinkling of rolled oats for texture.

- Try adding a scoop of your favourite protein powder to the mix for additional protein.

This Berry Burst Oat Smoothie is a delicious blend of fruity sweetness and nutty richness, delivering a nutritious and complete start to your day. The mix of berries and oats gives prolonged energy and a boost of nutrients, making it a perfect choice for people searching for a healthy breakfast or snack alternative.

Green Goddess Smoothie

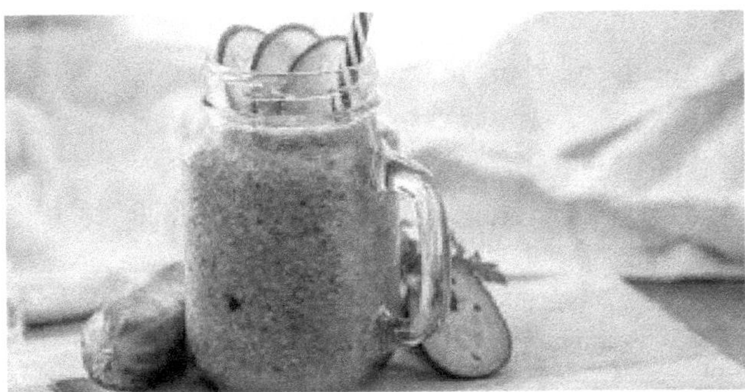

Embrace the vivid world of green deliciousness with our Green Goddess Smoothie. Packed with bright greens, creamy avocado, and the natural sweetness of banana, this smoothie is a pleasant way to launch your day with a blast of nutrition and energy. Including coconut water and chia seeds provides additional hydration and a hint of texture, making it a healthy option for a refreshing breakfast or a post-workout treat.

Ingredients:

- 1 cup fresh spinach leaves
- 1 cup kale leaves (stems removed)
- ½ ripe avocado, pitted and peeled
- One ripe banana
- 1 cup coconut water
- 1 tbsp chia seeds
- Ice cubes (optional)

Instructions:

Prepare the Ingredients:

- Wash the spinach, and kale leaves well.
- Remove the stems from the kale leaves and coarsely slice them.
- Cut the avocado in half, remove the pit, and scoop out the flesh.
- Peel the ripe banana and split it into bits.
- Measure out the coconut water and chia seeds.

Blend the Greens:

- Add the fresh spinach and cut kale leaves to your Vitamix mixer.

Creamy Avocado with Banana:

- Add the ripe avocado and banana pieces to the blender.

Add Liquid and Chia Seeds:

- Pour the coconut water and sprinkle the chia seeds over the remaining ingredients.

- Add a handful of ice cubes to the blender if you like a more relaxed texture.

Blend Until Smooth:

- Start mixing on low speed and gradually raise to high.
- Blend until the mixture is smooth and all the components are thoroughly combined.

Taste and Adjust:

- Add a banana or coconut water to taste the smoothie and adjust the sweetness or thickness.

Serve and Enjoy:

- Pour the Green Goddess Smoothie into glasses.
- Optionally, you may sprinkle a few additional chia seeds for added texture.

Quick Tip:

- Customize this smoothie by adding a tiny piece of ginger or a squeeze of lemon for an added flavour spike.

This Green Goddess Smoothie is a terrific way to integrate nutrient-rich leafy greens into your diet in a pleasant and accessible manner. Its refreshing flavour and creamy texture make it a perfect option for people wishing to improve their daily dose of vitamins, minerals, and antioxidants.

Peanut Butter Banana Power Shake

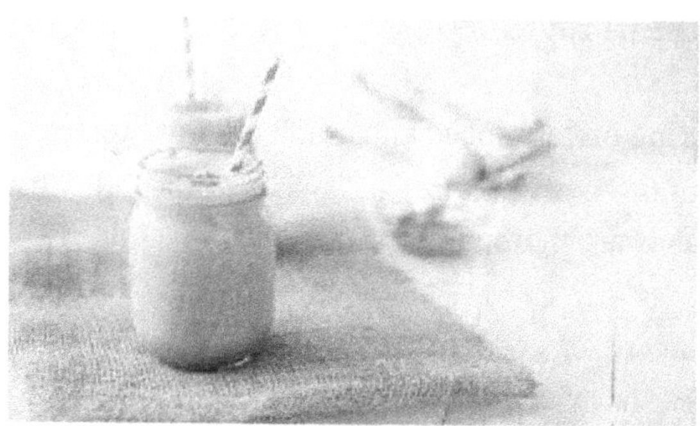

Get ready to power up your morning with the beautiful peanut butter and banana combo in this Peanut Butter Banana Power Shake. Packed with protein, healthy fats, and energy-boosting elements, this smoothie is tasty but also gratifying and nutritious. Whether you need a quick breakfast on the move or a post-workout refuel, this smoothie has got you covered.

Ingredients:

- Two ripe bananas
- Two tablespoons peanut butter (or nut butter of your choice)
- One scoop of chocolate protein powder
- 1 cup milk (dairy or plant-based)
- Handful of fresh spinach (optional, for additional greens)
- Ice cubes (optional)

- Peel the ripe bananas and split them into bits.
- Measure out the peanut butter, chocolate protein powder, and milk.

- Add the banana chunks, peanut butter, chocolate protein powder, and milk to your Vitamix blender.

- Add a handful of fresh spinach to the blender if you want to sneak in some greens.

- Try adding a few ice cubes to the recipe for a colder and thicker texture.

- Start mixing on low speed and gradually raise to high.
- Blend until the sauce is smooth and all the components are properly blended.

- Give the shake a taste and adjust the sweetness or thickness by adding additional banana or milk if required.

- Pour the Peanut Butter Banana Power Shake into a glass.
- Optionally, sprinkle a touch of more peanut butter on top for decoration.

- Enhance the shake's nutritional profile by adding a tablespoon of chia seeds or a handful of oats for added fibre.

This Peanut Butter Banana Power Shake is a terrific way to start your day with a protein-packed and tasty combination. The combination of banana and peanut butter produces carbs, healthy fats, and protein that may keep you nourished and motivated throughout the morning. Whether you're hitting the gym or confronting a hectic day, this drink will likely become your go-to breakfast pick.

Creamy Chia Pudding Smoothie

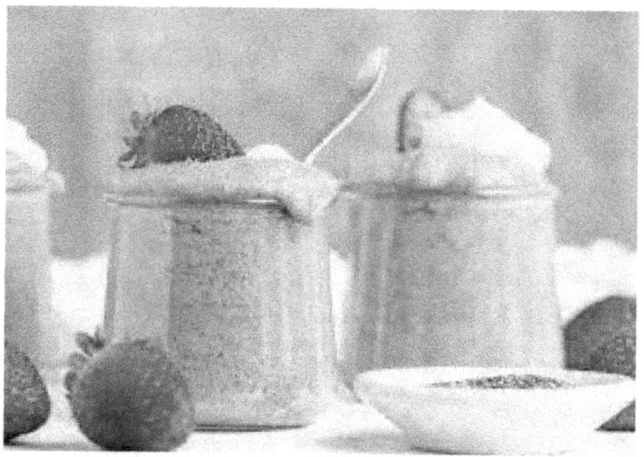

Combine the velvety richness of chia pudding with the ease of a smoothie in this Creamy Chia Pudding Smoothie. This unusual combination combines the health of chia seeds, almond milk, and a hint of sweetness to produce a lovely fusion of tastes and sensations. It's a fantastic way to experience the advantages of chia pudding while sipping on a pleasant and healthy smoothie.

For the Chia Pudding:

- ¼ cup chia seeds
- 1 cup almond milk (or milk of your choice)
- One tablespoon of honey or maple syrup
- ½ teaspoon vanilla extract For the Smoothie:
- One ripe banana
- ½ cup mixed berries (fresh or frozen)
- ½ cup almond milk (or milk of your choice)
- Ice cubes (optional)

Instructions:

Prepare the Chia Pudding:

- Combine the chia seeds, almond milk, honey or maple syrup, and vanilla extract in a dish.
- Stir carefully to ensure the chia seeds are uniformly dispersed.
- Place the Bowl in the refrigerator and let the mixture rest for at least 2 hours or overnight to let the chia seeds absorb the liquid and produce a pudding-like consistency.

Prepare the Smoothie:

Prepare the Ingredients:

- Peel the ripe banana and split it into bits.
- If using fresh berries, wash and remove any stems. If using frozen berries, there's no need to defrost them.
- Measure out the almond milk for the smoothie.

Blend the Smoothie Base:

- Add the ripe banana, mixed berries, and almond milk to your Vitamix mixer.

Blend Chia Pudding into Smoothie:

- Spoon the prepared chia pudding into the blender.

Optional: Add Ice:

- If you like a more astounding texture, add a handful of ice cubes to the blender.

Blend Until Smooth:

- Start mixing on low speed and gradually raise to high.
- Blend until all the ingredients are thoroughly blended and the smoothie is creamy.

Taste and Adjust:

- Give the smoothie a taste and adjust the sweetness or thickness by adding additional honey, banana, or almond milk as desired.

Serve and Enjoy:

- Pour the Creamy Chia Pudding Smoothie into glasses.
- You may top the smoothie with more chia pudding if desired.

- Customize the smoothie by adding a dollop of nut butter or sprinkling your favourite seeds.

This Creamy Chia Pudding Smoothie is a beautiful mix of chia pudding's pleasing texture with the refreshing flavour of a smoothie. It's a terrific way to include the benefits of chia seeds, which are high in fibre and omega-3 fatty acids, into your daily routine. Enjoy the unusual blend of tastes and textures as you sip your way to a healthful start to the day.

Cinnamon Roll Smoothie Bowl

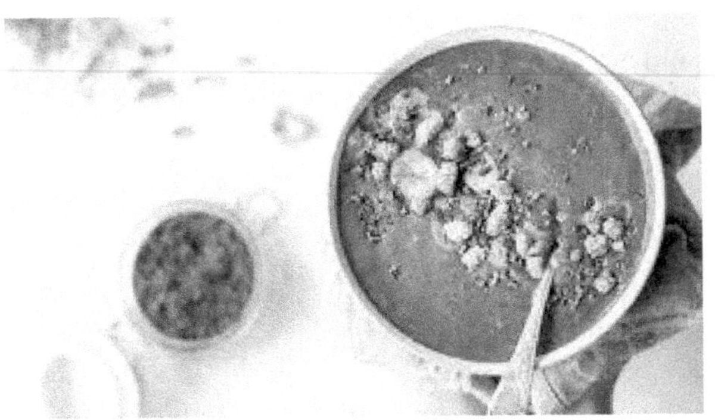

Indulge in the comforting tastes of a cinnamon bun healthily with our Cinnamon Bun Smoothie Bowl. Packed with the warmth of cinnamon, the creaminess of banana, and the heartiness of oats, this smoothie bowl captures the spirit of a traditional delight while giving a healthful and fulfilling morning choice.

Ingredients:

For the Smoothie Base:

- Two ripe bananas
- ½ cup rolled oats
- One teaspoon of ground cinnamon
- ½ teaspoon vanilla extract
- 1 cup milk (dairy or plant-based)
- Ice cubes (optional)

For Toppings:

- Chopped nuts (such as almonds, walnuts, or pecans)
- Drizzle honey or maple syrup
- Ground cinnamon
- Sliced bananas
- Dried fruits (such as raisins or cranberries)
- Granola

Instructions:

Prepare the Ingredients:

- Peel the ripe bananas and split them into bits.
- Measure out the rolled oats, ground cinnamon, vanilla essence, and milk.

Blend the Smoothie Base:

- Add the ripe banana chunks, rolled oats, ground cinnamon, vanilla essence, and milk to your Vitamix blender.

Optional: Add Ice:

- Add a few ice cubes to the blender if you like a colder and thicker texture.

Blend Until Smooth:

- Start mixing on low speed and gradually raise to high.
- Blend until all the components are thoroughly blended and the product is smooth.

Taste and Adjust:

- Give the smoothie a taste and adjust the sweetness or thickness by adding banana or milk.

Pour into a Bowl:

- Pour the smoothie into a bowl, forming a foundation for your toppings.

Add Toppings:

- Sprinkle chopped nuts, a drizzle of honey or maple syrup, a sprinkle of ground cinnamon, sliced bananas, dried fruits, and granola over the smoothie.

Enjoy:

- Use a spoon to delve into your Cinnamon Roll Smoothie Bowl, ensuring you receive a taste of the tasty smoothie base and the pleasant crunch of the toppings.

Quick Tip:

- Experiment with various toppings to customize your bowls, such as shredded coconut, chocolate nibs, or fresh berries.

This Cinnamon Roll Smoothie Bowl gives the familiar flavour of a cinnamon roll while offering a wholesome and energy-boosting breakfast. It's a terrific way to enrich your morning routine with the soothing scent and taste of cinnamon, producing a pleasant breakfast experience that's both gratifying and healthful.

Protein-Packed Coffee Smoothie

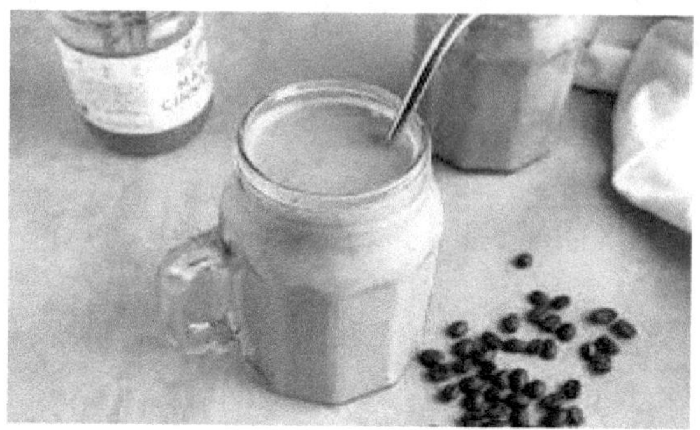

Combine the rich and stimulating aromas of coffee with the protein-packed deliciousness of a smoothie in this Protein-Packed Coffee Smoothie. Whether you're searching for a morning pick-me-up or a post-workout refill, this smoothie offers continuous energy and protein benefits to power through your day.

Ingredients:

- 1 cup cold brew coffee (or chilled strong coffee)
- One scoop of chocolate protein powder (or the flavour of your choice)
- One ripe banana
- ½ cup milk (dairy or plant-based)
- ¼ cup Greek yogurt
- One tablespoon of honey or maple syrup (optional for extra sweetness)
- Ice cubes (optional)

Prepare the Ingredients:

- Brew a cup of cold brew coffee and let it cool, or use cooled strong coffee.
- Peel the ripe banana and split it into bits.
- Measure out the chocolate protein powder, milk, Greek yogurt, and sweetener (if using).

Blend the Coffee Base:

- Add the cold brew coffee, chocolate protein powder, ripe banana, milk, Greek yogurt, and sweetener (if using) to your Vitamix blender.

Optional: Add Ice:

- Add a handful of ice cubes to the blender if you like a colder and thicker texture.

Blend Until Smooth:

- Start mixing on low speed and gradually raise to high.
- Blend until the mixture is smooth and fully incorporated.

Taste and Adjust:

- Give the smoothie a taste and adjust the sweetness or thickness by adding additional banana, milk, or sweetener as desired.

Serve and Enjoy:

- Pour the Protein-Packed Coffee Smoothie into a glass.
- You may also add a dab of chocolate syrup for extra enjoyment.

- Customize the smoothie by adding a dash of cinnamon, a tablespoon of nut butter, or a splash of vanilla extract.

This Protein-Packed Coffee Smoothie gives the pleasant mix of coffee's robust tastes and the protein boost required to power your day. It's a beautiful alternative for people searching for an effective and enjoyable method to include protein into their regimen while enjoying the stimulating benefits of coffee. This smoothie will delight your taste buds and motivate you whether drinking it for breakfast or as a mid-day snack.

Mango-Coconut Chia Parfait

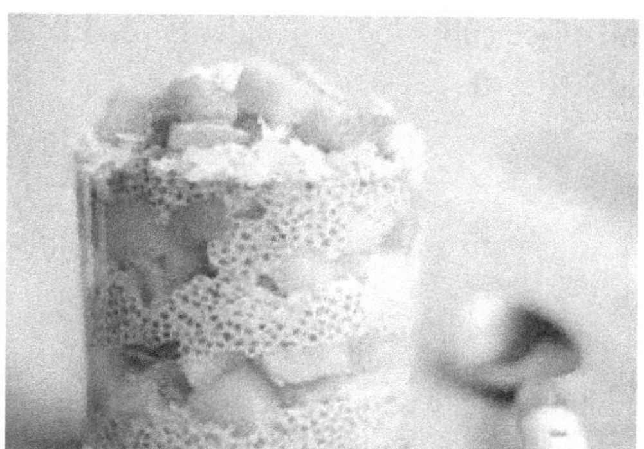

Indulge in a tropical pleasure with our Mango-Coconut Chia Parfait. Combining the creamy deliciousness of coconut milk with the sweetness of ripe mango and the texture of chia seeds, this parfait gives a balanced and delectable dessert-inspired breakfast. Layered to perfection, it's aesthetically stunning and a healthful and pleasant way to start your day.

Ingredients:

For the Chia Pudding:

- ¼ cup chia seeds
- 1 cup coconut milk (full-fat or mild)
- One tablespoon of honey or maple syrup
- ½ teaspoon vanilla extract

For the Mango Layer:

One ripe mango, peeled and diced. For Assembly:

- Chopped nuts (such as almonds or cashews)
- Toasted coconut flakes
- Fresh mint leaves (for garnish)

Instructions:

Prepare the Chia Pudding:

- Combine the chia seeds, coconut milk, honey or maple syrup, and vanilla extract in a dish.
- Stir carefully to ensure the chia seeds are uniformly dispersed.
- Place the Bowl in the refrigerator and let the mixture rest for at least 2 hours or overnight to let the chia seeds absorb the liquid and produce a pudding-like consistency.

Assemble the Mango-Coconut Chia Parfait:

Prepare the Ingredients:

- Peel and dice the ripe mango.

- Optionally, toast the coconut flakes in a dry skillet until gently brown for extra flavour and crunch.

Layer the Parfait:

- Start by spooning a layer of chia pudding into the bottom of a glass or container.
- Add a layer of chopped mango on top of the chia pudding.

Repeat the Layers:

- Add another layer of chia pudding.
- Top with another layer of chopped mango.

Finish with Toppings:

- Sprinkle chopped nuts and toasted coconut flakes over the top layer.
- Garnish with fresh mint leaves for a blast of colour and scent.

Serve and Enjoy:

- Use a large spoon to savour the chia pudding and mango layers, together with the delicious crunch of almonds and coconut.

Quick Tip:

- Customize your parfait by adding granola, yogurt, or extra fruit layers.

This Mango-Coconut Chia Parfait delivers a blend of creamy coconut, juicy mango, and the texture of chia seeds in an aesthetically attractive presentation. It's a great way to savour the tastes of the tropics while benefitting from the nutritious benefits of chia seeds and coconut milk. Whether you're eating it as a morning treat or a delicious dessert, this parfait is guaranteed to transport you to a sunny paradise with every mouthful.

Apple Pie Smoothie

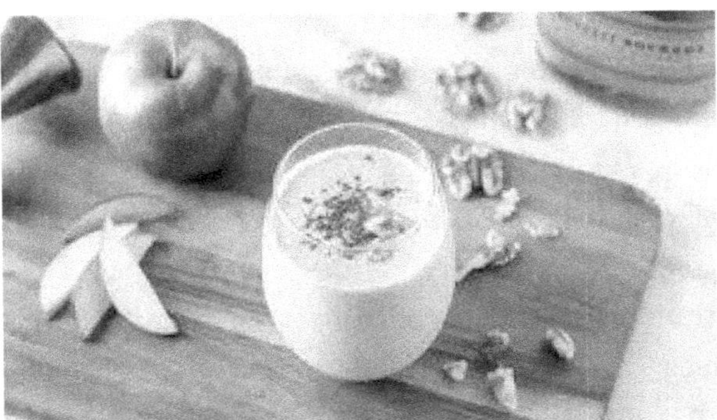

Experience the soothing tastes of apple pie in a simple and healthful Apple Pie Smoothie. This mix captures the essence of this famous dish with the sweetness of apples, the warmth of cinnamon, and a trace of nutmeg. It's a great way to revel in the aromas of autumn while enjoying the advantages of a nutritious and refreshing meal.

Ingredients:

- Two medium apples, cored and diced (leave the peel on for additional fibre)
- ½ cup rolled oats
- One teaspoon of ground cinnamon
- ¼ teaspoon ground nutmeg
- 1 cup milk (dairy or plant-based)
- One tablespoon almond butter (or nut butter of your choice)
- One tablespoon of honey or maple syrup
- Ice cubes (optional)

Instructions:

Prepare the Ingredients:
- Wash, core, and cut the apples. Leaving the skin on adds texture and fibre.
- Measure out the rolled oats, ground cinnamon, ground nutmeg, milk, almond butter, and sweetener.

Blend the Apple Pie Base:
- Add the diced apples, rolled oats, cinnamon, ground nutmeg, milk, almond butter, and sweetener to your Vitamix mixer.

Optional: Add Ice:
- Add a handful of ice cubes to the blender for a colder and thicker texture.

Blend Until Smooth:
- Start mixing on low speed and gradually raise to high.
- Blend until all the components are thoroughly blended and the product is smooth.

Taste and Adjust:
- Add apple, honey, or milk as desired to give the smoothie a taste and adjust the sweetness or thickness.

Serve and Enjoy:
- Pour the Apple Pie Smoothie into glasses.
- You may add put a pinch of ground cinnamon on top for decoration.

Quick Tip:
- For increased protein, try adding a scoop of vanilla or cinnamon-flavoured protein powder to the mix.

This Apple Pie Smoothie gives the pleasant and nostalgic flavour of apple pie while delivering a healthy start to your day. It's a lovely way to savour the tastes of autumn without the additional sweets and calories of conventional desserts. Sip on this smoothie and taste the mix of apples, spices, and creamy almond butter in a wonderfully balanced blend.

Blueberry Almond Breakfast Bowl

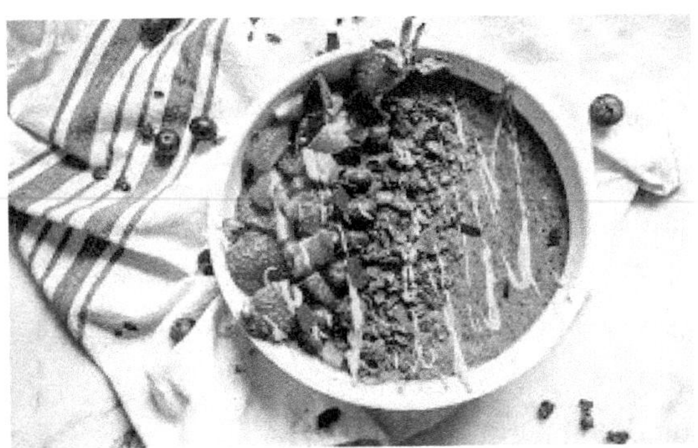

Elevate your morning with the rich taste of blueberries and the delicious crunch of almonds in this Blueberry Almond Morning Bowl. Packed with antioxidants, healthy fats, and natural sweetness, this Bowl delivers a nourishing and delightful way to begin your day on a healthful note.

Ingredients:

- 1 cup blueberries (fresh or frozen)
- ½ cup almond milk (or milk of your choice)
- ½ cup Greek yogurt
- Handful of almonds, chopped

- Drizzle honey or maple syrup
- Fresh blueberries (for topping)
- Granola (for topping)
- Chia seeds (for topping)

Instructions:

Prepare the Ingredients:

- If using frozen blueberries, let them defrost slightly.
- Measure out the almond milk, Greek yogurt, chopped almonds, honey or maple syrup, fresh blueberries, granola, and chia seeds.

Blend the Blueberry Base:

- Add the blueberries, almond milk, and Greek yogurt to your Vitamix blender.

Blend Until Smooth:

- Start mixing on low speed and gradually raise to high.
- Blend until the mixture is smooth and the blueberries are thoroughly integrated.

Assemble the Breakfast Bowl:

- Pour the blueberry mixture into a bowl.

Add Toppings:

- Sprinkle the chopped almonds over the blueberry foundation.
- Drizzle honey or maple syrup for extra sweetness.
- Add a handful of fresh blueberries for texture and colour.
- Sprinkle granola and chia seeds for crunch and extra nutrients.

- Use a spoon to delve into your Blueberry Almond Breakfast Bowl, savouring the creamy blueberry base and the lovely blend of toppings.

- Feel free to personalize your Bowl with additional favourite toppings, such as shredded coconut, sliced bananas, or dried fruits.

This Blueberry Almond Breakfast Bowl is a terrific way to embrace the antioxidants and minerals found in blueberries while enjoying the pleasant crunch of almonds and other healthy toppings. Its delicious taste and textures make it a perfect choice for people wishing to start their day with a balanced and aesthetically pleasing breakfast.

CHAPTER THREE

Fresh and Vibrant Soups

Creamy Tomato Basil Soup

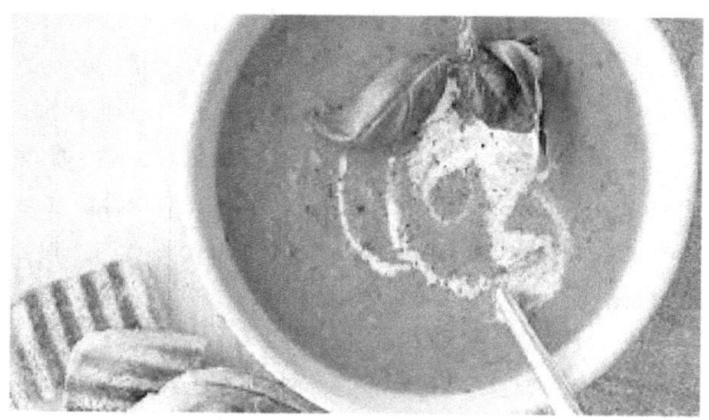

This easy and tasty recipe includes the soothing tastes of a traditional Creamy Tomato Basil Soup. Using fresh tomatoes and aromatic basil, this soup is an excellent blend of rich creaminess and bright tanginess. Enjoy it as a cozy meal, or combine it with crusty toast for a fulfilling lunch or supper.

Ingredients:

- Four big tomatoes, cored and quartered
- One onion, chopped
- Three cloves garlic, minced
- 2 cups vegetable broth
- ½ cup heavy cream (or coconut milk for a dairy-free alternative)

- ¼ cup fresh basil leaves
- Two tablespoons of olive oil
- Salt and pepper to taste
- Optional toppings: more basil leaves, a sprinkle of olive oil, croutons

Instructions:

Sauté Aromatics:

- In a large saucepan, heat the olive oil over medium heat.
- Add the diced onion and minced garlic. Sauté until the onion is transparent and aromatic.

Add Tomatoes:

- Add the quartered tomatoes to the saucepan. Cook for a few minutes until the tomatoes start to soften.

Simmer and Blend:

- Pour in the veggie broth and bring the mixture to a low boil. Cook for around 15-20 minutes until the tomatoes are thoroughly softened.
- Carefully put the mixture in your Vitamix blender.

Blend Until Smooth:

- Add the fresh basil leaves and blend on high until the mixture is smooth and creamy.

Return to Pot:

- Pour the combined mixture back into the saucepan.

Add Cream:

- Stir in the heavy cream (coconut milk) and boil the soup over low heat until warm. Do not let it boil.

- Season the soup with salt and pepper to taste.
- Ladle the Creamy Tomato Basil Soup into bowls.

- Garnish with more fresh basil leaves, a drizzle of olive oil, or croutons if preferred.

- Enjoy your Creamy Tomato Basil Soup with crusty bread for dipping.

- To increase the taste, roast the tomatoes in the oven before putting them in the soup.

This Creamy Tomato Basil Soup combines the soothing flavour of tomatoes and the fragrant scent of basil. It's a classic favourite that can be prepared quickly in your Vitamix blender, offering a bowl of comfort and pleasure with every mouthful.

Green Pea and Mint Soup

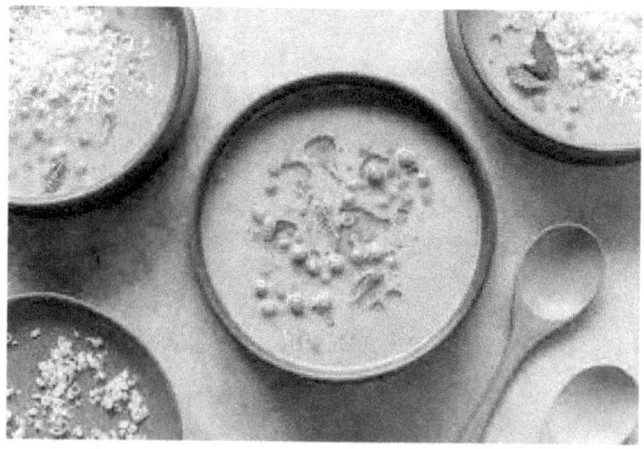

Experience the fresh and vivid mix of green peas and mint in this delectable Green Pea and Mint Soup. With its brilliant colour and refreshing taste, this soup is a fantastic option for a light and healthy dinner. Serve it hot or cold, depending on the season and your inclination.

- 2 cups fresh or frozen green peas
- One small onion, chopped
- Two cloves garlic, minced
- 4 cups vegetable broth
- ¼ cup fresh mint leaves
- Two tablespoons of olive oil
- Salt and pepper to taste
- Optional toppings: yogurt drizzle, additional mint leaves, croutons

- In a large saucepan, heat the olive oil over medium heat.
- Add the diced onion and minced garlic. Sauté until the onion is transparent and aromatic.

- Add the green peas to the saucepan and boil for a few minutes.
- Pour in the veggie broth and bring the mixture to a boil. Let it simmer for 10-15 minutes until the peas are soft.

Blend the Soup:

- Carefully pour the pea and broth mixture into your Vitamix blender.

Add Mint:

- Add the fresh mint leaves to the blender.

Blend Until Smooth:

- Blend on high until the soup is smooth and creamy.

Return to Pot:

- Pour the pureed soup back into the pot.

Season and Serve:

- Season the soup with salt and pepper to taste.

Reheat and Serve:

- Heat the soup over low heat until warmed through.

Serve with Toppings:

- Ladle the Green Pea and Mint Soup into dishes.
- Drizzle with a bit of yogurt for additional creaminess.
- Garnish with more mint leaves and croutons if preferred.

Enjoy Hot or Cold:

- This soup may be served hot or cold, depending on your choice.

This Green Pea and Mint Soup blasts freshness and a lovely combination of flavours. The sweetness of peas and the fragrant scent of mint create a harmonic balance that's both calming and stimulating. Whether consumed as a light lunch or a refreshing appetizer, this soup will liven up your lunchtime.

Roasted Red Pepper Soup

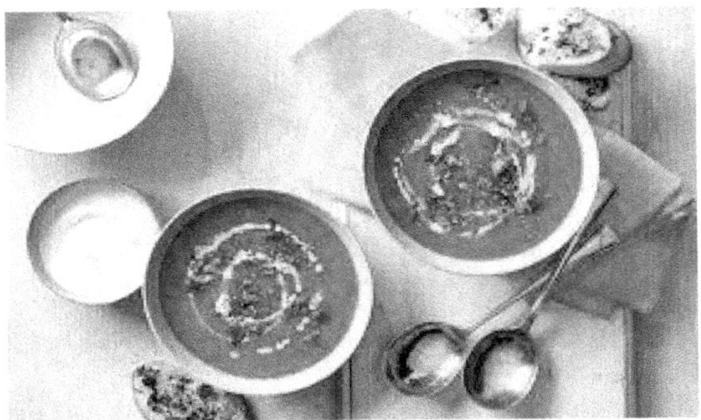

Savour the smoky-sweet tastes of roasted red peppers in this rich and cozy Roasted Red Pepper Soup. Adding onions, garlic, and warming spices gives this soup a snug and tasty alternative for a fulfilling supper.

Ingredients:

- Four big red bell peppers
- One onion, chopped
- Three cloves garlic, minced
- 2 cups vegetable broth
- ½ cup heavy cream (or coconut milk for a dairy-free alternative)
- Two tablespoons of olive oil
- One teaspoon of smoked paprika
- Salt and pepper to taste
- Optional toppings: fresh parsley, a sprinkle of olive oil, sour cream or yogurt

Instructions:

Roast the Red Peppers:

- Preheat your oven's broiler. Place the red bell peppers on a baking pan and sprinkle with olive oil.
- Broil the peppers, rotating periodically, until the skin is browned and blistered. This should take 10-15 minutes.
- Remove the peppers from the oven and transfer them to a bowl. Cover the Bowl with plastic wrap or a cover and let the peppers steam for approximately 10 minutes. This will make it simpler to peel the skins.

Peel and Prep:

- Once the peppers are cool enough to handle, peel off the charred skins, remove the stems and seeds, and coarsely cut the meat.

Sauté Aromatics:

- In a large saucepan, heat the olive oil over medium heat.
- Add the diced onion and minced garlic. Sauté until the onion is transparent and aromatic.

Blend the Red Pepper Base:

- Add the roasted red pepper pieces to the saucepan.

Add Broth and Spices:

- Pour the vegetable broth and add the smoked paprika, salt, and pepper.
- Let the mixture boil for around 10 minutes.

Blend Until Smooth:

- Carefully put the mixture in your Vitamix blender.

- Blend on high until the soup is creamy and silky.
- Pour the pureed soup back into the pot.

- Stir in the heavy cream (coconut milk) and boil the soup over low heat until warm. Do not let it boil.

- Season the soup with extra salt and pepper if required.

- Ladle the Roasted Red Pepper Soup into bowls.
- Garnish with fresh parsley, a drizzle of olive oil, or a dollop of sour cream or yogurt if preferred.

This Roasted Red Pepper Soup captures roasted red peppers' rich and smokey taste while giving a silky texture and soothing flavours. It's a flexible choice that can be eaten independently or with your favourite side dishes. The blend of sweetness and smokiness makes it a pleasant option for any meal.

Carrot Ginger Soup

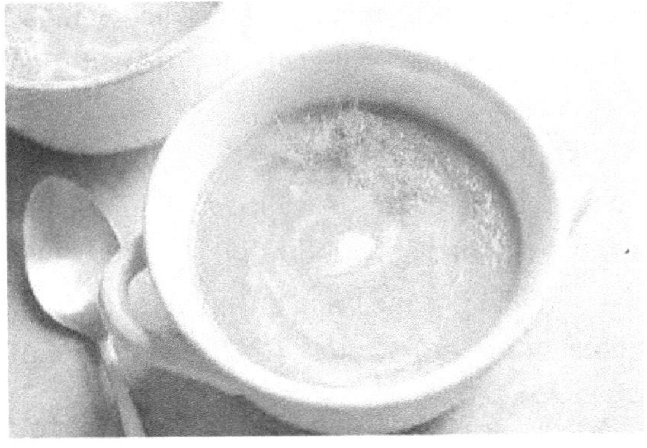

Embrace the warm and soothing tastes of carrots and ginger in this delectable Carrot Ginger Soup. With its brilliant colour and spicy bite, this soup is healthy and exhilarating, making it a fantastic option for a warm supper.

Ingredients:

- 4 cups carrots, peeled and diced
- One onion, chopped two cloves garlic, minced one tablespoon fresh ginger, minced
- 4 cups vegetable broth
- ½ cup coconut milk (or cream for additional richness)
- Two tablespoons of olive oil
- Salt and pepper to taste
- Optional toppings: minced fresh parsley, a drizzle of coconut milk, roasted pumpkin seeds

Instructions:

Sauté Aromatics:

- In a large saucepan, heat the olive oil over medium heat.
- Add the chopped onion, minced garlic, and minced ginger. Sauté until the onion is transparent and aromatic.

Add Carrots and Broth:

- Add the chopped carrots to the saucepan and simmer for a few minutes, stirring periodically.
- Pour in the veggie broth and bring the mixture to a boil. Let it simmer for approximately 20-25 minutes until the carrots are soft.

Blend the Soup:

- Carefully transfer the cooked carrot mixture to your Vitamix blender.

Blend Until Smooth:

- Blend on high until the soup is smooth and creamy.

Return to Pot:

- Pour the pureed soup back into the pot.

Add Coconut Milk:

- Stir in the coconut milk (or cream) to give richness and creaminess to the soup.

Season and Reheat:

- Season the soup with salt and pepper to taste.
- Heat the soup over low heat until warmed through. Do not let it boil.

Serve with Toppings:

- Ladle the Carrot Ginger Soup into bowls.
- Drizzle with a touch of coconut milk for additional richness.
- Sprinkle chopped fresh parsley and roasted pumpkin seeds on top if preferred.

Enjoy the Flavors:

- Savour the soothing tastes of carrots and ginger in every mouthful.

Quick Tip:

- For an added depth of flavour, you may sauté the carrots quickly in the saucepan before adding the aromatics.

This Carrot Ginger Soup delivers a lovely blend of sweetness and spicy warmth. The pairing of carrots and ginger provides a harmonic balance that's both calming and refreshing. Whether consumed as a light lunch or as part of a heartier supper, this soup will brighten your taste senses and fulfill your yearning for comfort.

Cucumber Gazpacho

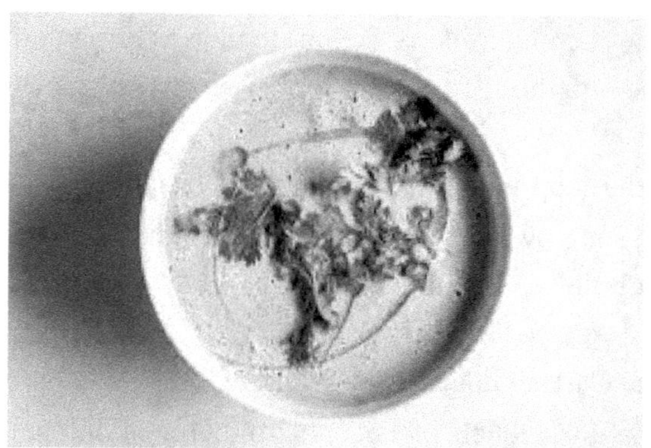

Indulge in the pleasant scents of summer with this cool and vivid Cucumber Gazpacho. Bursting with the chill of cucumbers, the sharpness of tomatoes, and the zing of bell peppers, this soup is a fantastic way to avoid the heat while enjoying a healthy and delectable dinner.

Ingredients:

- Two big cucumbers peeled and cut
- 2 cups ripe tomatoes, chopped one red bell pepper, chopped one small red onion, chopped two cloves garlic, minced ¼ cup fresh cilantro or parsley, chopped three tablespoons olive oil

- Two teaspoons of red wine vinegar
- 2 cups vegetable broth
- Salt and pepper to taste
- Optional toppings: sliced cucumber, chopped herbs, croutons

Instructions:

Blend the Vegetables:

- Add the diced cucumbers, tomatoes, red bell pepper, red onion, minced garlic, and fresh cilantro or parsley in your Vitamix blender.

Blend Until Smooth:

- Blend on high until the mixture is fully incorporated and achieves a smooth consistency.

Add Olive Oil and Vinegar:

- With the blender running low speed, carefully drip in the olive oil and red wine vinegar until well mixed.

Add Vegetable Broth:

- Pour the vegetable broth and continue mixing until the soup is thoroughly blended.

Season and Chill:

- Season the soup with salt and pepper to taste.
- Transfer the combined mixture to a bowl and refrigerate for at least 1 hour to enable the flavours to merge and the soup to be cold.

Serve Chilled:

- Ladle the cooled Cucumber Gazpacho into bowls.

- Garnish with sliced cucumber, chopped herbs, and croutons if preferred.

- Adjust the consistency by adding extra vegetable broth if you like a thinner soup.

This Cucumber Gazpacho is a light and energizing alternative for warm days. Its crisp and refreshing taste makes it a fantastic way to appreciate the richness of summer fruit. Whether searching for a light appetizer or a vital and fulfilling main meal, this gazpacho will likely become a staple in your summer menu.

Spinach and Avocado Soup

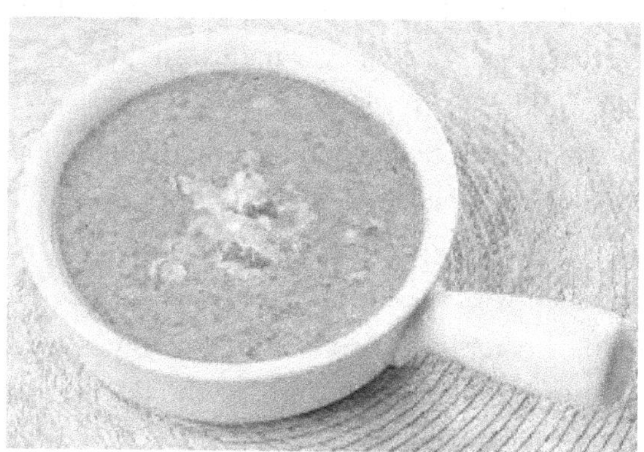

Embrace the richness of greens and the smoothness of avocado in this healthy Spinach and Avocado Soup. Packed with nutrients and colourful tastes, this soup is delicious and refreshing, making it a terrific option for a light and balanced supper.

4 cups fresh spinach leaves, cleaned and stems removed

- Two ripe avocados peeled and pitted
- One small onion, chopped
- Two cloves garlic, minced
- 4 cups vegetable broth
- ½ cup Greek yogurt (or coconut yogurt for a dairy-free alternative)
- Juice of 1 lemon
- Two tablespoons of olive oil
- Salt and pepper to taste
- Optional toppings: chopped fresh herbs, a spray of olive oil, pumpkin seeds

Instructions:

Sauté Aromatics:

- In a large saucepan, heat the olive oil over medium heat.
- Add the diced onion and minced garlic. Sauté until the onion is transparent and aromatic.

Add Spinach and Broth:

- Add the fresh spinach leaves to the saucepan and simmer for a few minutes until wilted.
- Pour in the veggie broth and bring the mixture to a boil. Let it cook for approximately 10 minutes.

Blend the Spinach Base:

- Carefully transfer the cooked spinach mixture to your Vitamix blender.

- Add the peeled and pitted avocados to the blender.
- Add the Greek yogurt (or coconut yogurt) and lemon juice.

Blend Until Smooth:

- Blend on high until the mixture is smooth and creamy.

Return to Pot:

- Pour the combined mixture back into the saucepan.

Season and Reheat:

Season the soup with salt and pepper to taste.

- Heat the soup over low heat until warmed through. Do not let it boil.

Serve with Toppings:

- Ladle the Spinach and Avocado Soup into dishes.
- Garnish with chopped fresh herbs, a sprinkle of olive oil, and pumpkin seeds if preferred.

Enjoy the Creaminess:

- Savour the creamy smoothness of avocado and the freshness of spinach in each mouthful.

Quick Tip:

- Add a handful of fresh mint or basil leaves to the blender for an added blast of freshness.

This Spinach and Avocado Soup delivers a delicious combination of creamy and vivid tastes. Its nutrient-packed components make it a terrific way to add greens to your diet while having a tasty and fulfilling dinner. This soup will leave you feeling filled and invigorated, whether savoured as a light lunch or a cozy supper.

Sweet Potato Curry Soup

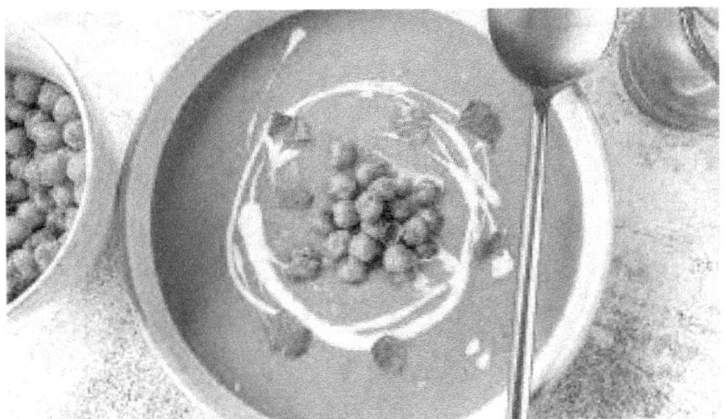

Experience the cozy combination of sweet potatoes and fragrant curry spices in this tasty and hearty Sweet Potato Curry Soup. With its rich and warming taste, this soup is a terrific option for a fulfilling supper that's both nutritional and soothing.

Ingredients:

- Two big sweet potatoes, peeled and sliced
- One onion, chopped three cloves garlic, minced
- One tablespoon of fresh ginger, minced
- One tablespoon of curry powder
- ½ teaspoon ground turmeric
- 4 cups vegetable broth
- 1 cup coconut milk (full-fat or mild)
- Two tablespoons of olive oil
- Salt and pepper to taste
- Optional toppings: chopped cilantro, a sprinkle of coconut milk, roasted cashews

Sauté Aromatics:

- In a large saucepan, heat the olive oil over medium heat.
- Add the chopped onion, minced garlic, and minced ginger. Sauté until the onion is transparent and aromatic.

Add Spices:

- Add the curry powder and ground turmeric to the saucepan. Stir well to coat the aromatics with the spices.

Add Sweet Potatoes and Broth:

- Add the chopped sweet potatoes to the saucepan and simmer for a few minutes, stirring periodically.
- Pour in the veggie broth and bring the mixture to a boil. Let everything stew for approximately 20-25 minutes until the sweet potatoes are soft.

Blend the Soup:

- Carefully transfer the cooked sweet potato mixture to your Vitamix blender.

Blend Until Smooth:

- Blend on high until the soup is creamy and silky.

Return to Pot:

- Pour the pureed soup back into the pot.

Add Coconut Milk:

- Stir in the coconut milk to give creaminess and richness to the soup.

-
- Season the soup with salt and pepper to taste.
- Heat the soup over low heat until warmed through. Do not let it boil.

- Ladle the Sweet Potato Curry Soup into bowls.
- Drizzle with a touch of coconut milk for additional richness.
- Sprinkle chopped cilantro and roasted cashews on top if desired.

- Savour the warm and savoury blend of sweet potatoes with curry spices.

This Sweet Potato Curry Soup brings together sweet potatoes' heartiness and curry spices' fragrant richness. Its velvety texture and warming taste make it a soothing option for a hearty supper. Whether served on its own or combined with your favourite bread or rice, this soup is guaranteed to fulfill your demands for comfort and taste.

Cold Zucchini and Dill Soup

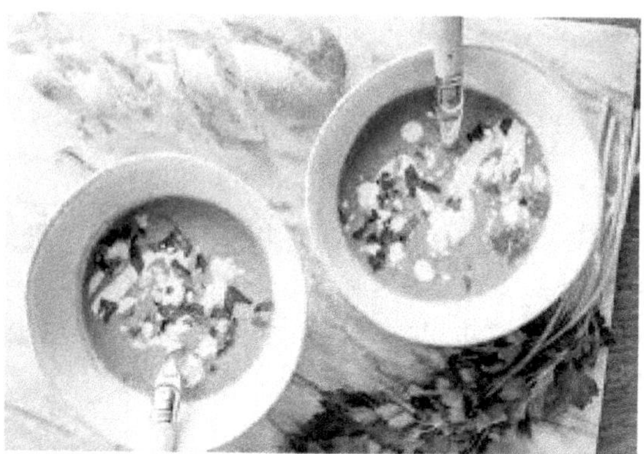

Experience the pleasant tastes of summer with this cooled and herb-infused Cold Zucchini and Dill Soup. Made with fresh zucchini and aromatic dill, this soup is a fantastic way to cool down on a hot day while enjoying a light and refreshing lunch.

Ingredients:

- Four medium zucchinis, chopped one small onion, chopped two cloves garlic, minced
- 1/4 cup fresh dill, chopped 4 cups vegetable broth
- 1 cup plain yogurt (Greek or regular)
- Two tablespoons of olive oil
- Juice of 1 lemon
- Salt and pepper to taste
- Optional toppings: chopped fresh dill, a sprinkle of olive oil, yogurt dollop

Sauté Aromatics:

- In a large saucepan, heat the olive oil over medium heat.
- Add the diced onion and minced garlic. Sauté until the onion is transparent and aromatic.

Add Zucchini and Broth:

- Add the chopped zucchini to the saucepan and simmer for a few minutes until slightly softened.
- Pour in the veggie broth and bring the mixture to a boil. Let it cook for approximately 10 minutes.

Blend the Zucchini Base:

- Carefully put the cooked zucchini mixture into your Vitamix blender.

Add Dill and Yogurt:

- Add the chopped dill and plain yogurt to the blender.
- Squeeze in the juice of one lemon.

Blend Until Smooth:

- Blend on high until the mixture is fully incorporated and achieves a smooth consistency.

Return to Pot:

- Pour the combined mixture back into the saucepan.

Season and Chill:

- Season the soup with salt and pepper to taste.
- Transfer the pot to the refrigerator and allow the soup to cold for at least 1 hour.

- Spoon the cooled Cold Zucchini and Dill Soup into dishes.

- Garnish with chopped fresh dill and a dab of olive oil if preferred.
- Optionally, add a dollop of yogurt to each dish.

- Enjoy the refreshing and energizing aromas of zucchini and dill in every mouthful.

This Cold Zucchini and Dill Soup is a lovely way to avoid the summer heat and enjoy the taste of fresh veggies. Its bright and herbaceous undertones make it a light and stimulating pick for a refreshing lunch. Whether consumed as an appetizer or a light main meal, this soup will leave you feeling relaxed and satiated.

Beet and Orange Soup

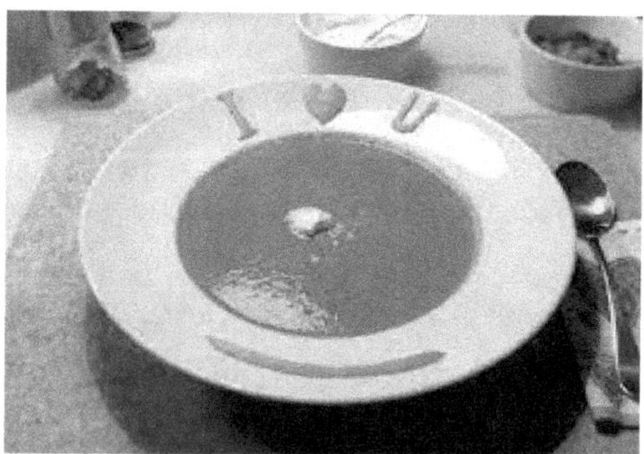

Discover the unusual combination of earthy beets and zesty oranges in this vivid and tangy Beet and Orange Soup. With its vibrant colours and refreshing aromas, this soup is a beautiful blend of sweet and spicy, making it a delicious option for a tasty and nutrient-packed supper.

Ingredients:

- Three big beets peeled and cut
- One onion, chopped two cloves garlic, minced
- Two oranges, zest and juice
- 4 cups vegetable broth
- 1/4 cup fresh orange juice
- Two tablespoons of olive oil
- Salt and pepper to taste
- Optional toppings: Greek yogurt or sour cream, minced fresh herbs, orange zest

Instructions:

Sauté Aromatics:

- In a large saucepan, heat the olive oil over medium heat.
- Add the diced onion and minced garlic. Sauté until the onion is transparent and aromatic.

Add Beets and Broth:

- Add the chopped beets to the saucepan and simmer for a few minutes until slightly mushy.
- Pour in the veggie broth and bring the mixture to a boil. Let it simmer for approximately 20-25 minutes until the beets are soft.

Blend the Beet Base:

- Carefully transfer the cooked beet mixture to your Vitamix blender.

Add Orange Zest and Juice:

- Add the zest and juice of two oranges to the blender.

Blend Until Smooth:

- Blend on high until the mixture is fully incorporated and achieves a smooth consistency.

Return to Pot:

- Pour the combined mixture back into the saucepan.

Add Fresh Orange Juice:

- Stir in the extra ¼ cup of fresh orange juice.

Season and Reheat:

- Season the soup with salt and pepper to taste.
- Heat the soup over low heat until warmed through. Do not let it boil.

Serve with Toppings:

- Ladle the Beet and Orange Soup into dishes.
- Garnish with a dollop of Greek yogurt or sour cream, chopped fresh herbs, and a sprinkle of orange zest if preferred.

Enjoy the Vibrancy:

- Savour the vibrant and contrasting aromas of beets and oranges in each mouthful.

This Beet and Orange Soup brings together beets' natural sweetness and oranges' zesty brightness. The blend of tastes provides a delicate balance that's both refreshing and enjoyable. Whether served as a light beginning or as the main dish, this soup is guaranteed to dazzle with its brilliant colours and distinctive flavour.

Mushroom and Thyme Bisque

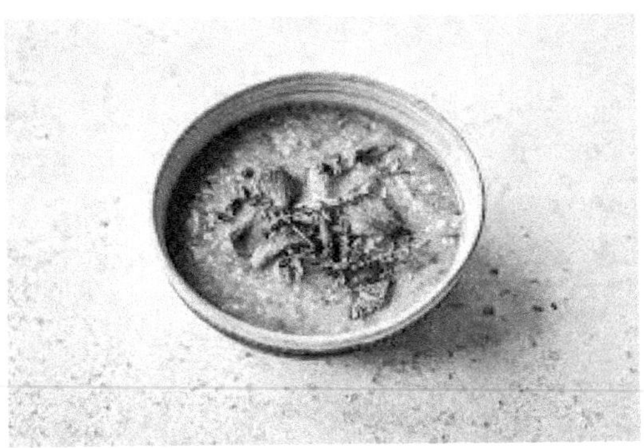

Indulge in the rich and velvety tastes of mushrooms and thyme in this luscious Mushroom and Thyme Bisque. With its creamy texture and aromatic richness, this soup is a fantastic option for a soothing and delicious supper.

Ingredients:

- 1 pound mushrooms, cleaned and sliced
- One onion, chopped
- Three cloves garlic, minced
- Two teaspoons fresh thyme leaves
- 4 cups vegetable broth
- 1 cup heavy cream (or coconut milk for a dairy-free alternative)

- Two tablespoons butter (or olive oil for a dairy-free option)
- Salt and pepper to taste
- Optional toppings: fresh thyme sprigs, a sprinkle of cream or olive oil, croutons

Instructions:

Sauté Aromatics:

- In a large saucepan, melt the butter over medium heat (or heat the olive oil for a dairy-free alternative).
- Add the diced onion and minced garlic. Sauté until the onion is transparent and aromatic.

Add Mushrooms and Thyme:

- Add the sliced mushrooms and fresh thyme leaves to the saucepan. Cook until the mushrooms are cooked and golden brown.

Blend the Mushroom Base:

- Carefully put the cooked mushroom mixture into your Vitamix blender.

Blend Until Smooth:

- Blend on high until the mixture is smooth and velvety.

Return to Pot:

- Pour the combined mixture back into the saucepan.

Add Cream:

- Stir in the heavy cream (or coconut milk) to give richness to the bisque.

Season and Reheat:

- Season the soup with salt and pepper to taste.

- Heat the soup over low heat until warmed through. Do not let it boil.

- Ladle the Mushroom and Thyme Bisque into bowls.
- Garnish with fresh thyme sprigs, cream or olive oil drizzle, and croutons if preferred.

- Enjoy the rich and savoury tastes of mushrooms and thyme in each mouthful.

- For an added depth of flavour, you may add a splash of white wine to the saucepan while sautéing the mushrooms.

This Mushroom and Thyme Bisque gives a beautiful and luxurious experience with its creamy texture and fragrant herbs. The richness of mushrooms and the floral scent of thyme combine to produce a soup that's excellent for special events or comfortable afternoons. Whether served as an appetizer or as the main meal, this bisque is guaranteed to fulfill your demands for comfort and taste.

CHAPTER FOUR

Delectable Dips and Spreads

Roasted Red Pepper Hummus

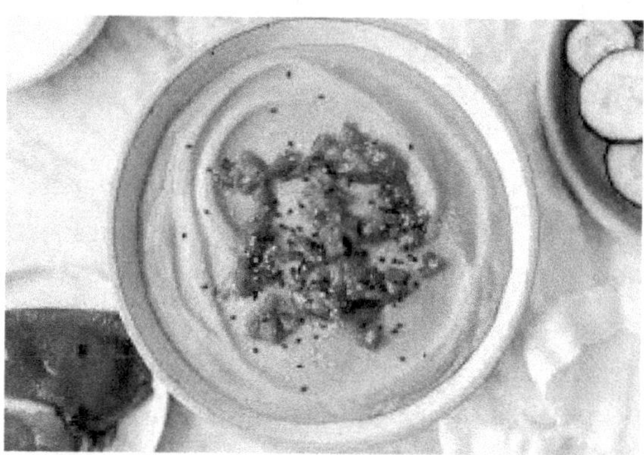

Indulge in the delicious aromas of this Roasted Red Pepper Hummus, a creamy and flavorful dip that's excellent for dipping veggies, pita bread, or using it as a spread. The roasted red peppers provide a hint of sweetness and brilliant colour to this traditional hummus recipe.

Ingredients:

- One can (15 oz) chickpeas, drained and rinsed
- ½ cup roasted red peppers (from a jar or handmade)
- ¼ cup tahini
- Two cloves garlic, minced
- Three tablespoons of lemon juice
- Two tablespoons of olive oil

- One teaspoon of ground cumin
- Salt and pepper to taste
- Optional toppings: additional roasted red pepper slices, chopped fresh parsley, a splash of olive oil

Instructions:

Blend Ingredients:

- Add drained chickpeas, roasted red peppers, tahini, minced garlic, lemon juice, olive oil, ground cumin, salt, and pepper in your Vitamix blender.

Blend Until Smooth:

- Start the blender on low speed and gradually raise it to high. Blend until the mixture is smooth and creamy.

Adjust Consistency:

- If the hummus is too thick, add a tablespoon or two of water while mixing to obtain your preferred consistency.

Taste and Adjust:

- Taste the hummus and adjust the spices, adding more lemon juice, salt, or cumin if required.

Serve and Garnish:

- Transfer the Roasted Red Pepper Hummus to a serving dish.
- Garnish with more strips of roasted red pepper, chopped fresh parsley, and a drizzle of olive oil if preferred.

Serve with Dippers:

- Serve the hummus with dippable things such as carrot sticks, cucumber slices, pita bread, or tortilla chips.

- Savour the sweet and savoury aromas of roasted red peppers and the creamy smoothness of the hummus.

This Roasted Red Pepper Hummus is a crowd-pleasing dip that's excellent for gatherings, parties, or just eating as a snack. The combination of chickpeas and roasted red peppers offers a beautiful mix of filling and tasty tastes. Customize the seasoning to your preference and enjoy the flexibility of this delicious dip.

Creamy Avocado Dip

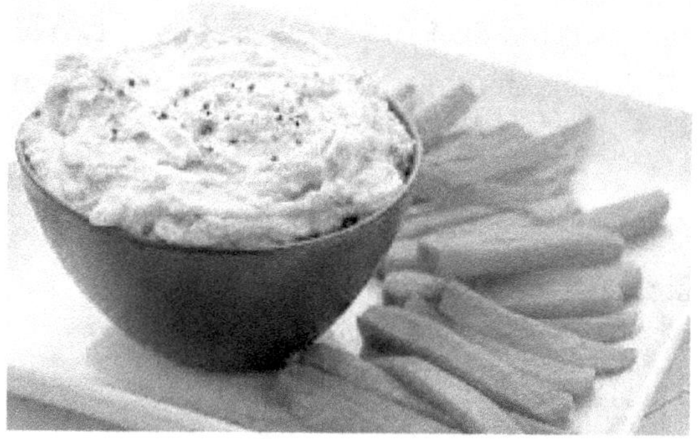

Enjoy the creamy deliciousness of avocados in this scrumptious Creamy Avocado Dip. Bursting with freshness and zesty tastes, this dip is excellent for dipping veggies, tortilla chips, or spread over toast for a fast and healthy snack.

Ingredients:

- Two ripe avocados peeled and pitted

- ¼ cup plain Greek yogurt
- Juice of 1 lime
- One clove of garlic, minced
- ¼ teaspoon ground cumin
- Salt and pepper to taste
- Optional toppings: chopped fresh cilantro, diced tomatoes, red onion, or jalapeño

Instructions:

Blend Avocado Mixture:

- Add the ripe avocados, plain Greek yogurt, lime juice, chopped garlic, ground cumin, salt, and pepper in your Vitamix blender.

Blend Until Creamy:

- Blend on low speed, gradually increasing to high, until the mixture is creamy and smooth.

Adjust Consistency:

- Add a tablespoon of water or extra yogurt to obtain your preferred consistency if the dip is too thick.

Taste and Adjust:

- Taste the dip and adjust the taste by adding additional lime juice, salt, or cumin if required.

Serve and Garnish:

- Transfer the Creamy Avocado Dip to a serving dish.

Garnish and Customize:

- Customize the dip by garnishing it with chopped fresh cilantro, diced tomatoes, red onion, or a dash of sliced jalapeño for extra spice.

- Serve the dip with a selection of dippers such as carrot sticks, bell pepper slices, cucumber rounds, or your favourite tortilla chips.

- Savour the velvety texture and zesty flavours of this delightful avocado dip.

This Creamy Avocado Dip is a flexible and healthful alternative for snacking or entertaining. The combination of avocados and Greek yogurt makes a rich and fulfilling dip that's not only delectable but also filled with healthy fats and protein. Whether eating it alone or using it as a spread, this dip will likely become a favourite.

Spinach and Artichoke Dip

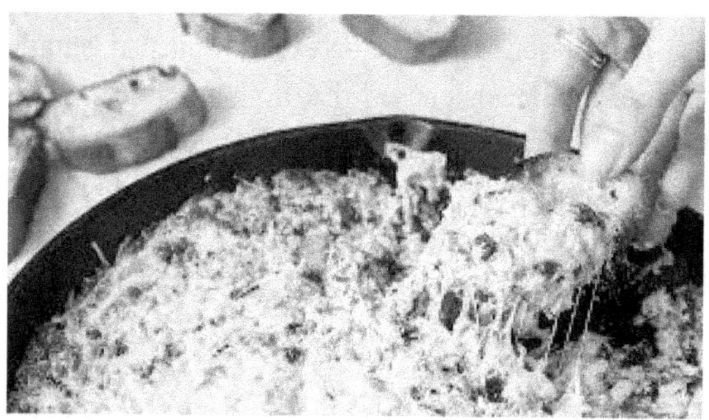

Indulge in the creamy and savoury pleasure of our traditional Spinach and Artichoke Dip. Made with sautéed spinach, marinated artichokes, and a cheesy base, this dip is excellent for parties, game nights, or just savouring as a soothing snack.

- 8 ounces fresh spinach, cleaned and chopped
- One can (14 oz) marinated artichoke hearts, drained and diced
- 1 cup cream cheese, softened
- ½ cup sour cream
- ½ cup mayonnaise
- 1 cup grated Parmesan cheese
- 1 cup shredded mozzarella cheese
- Two cloves garlic, minced
- ¼ teaspoon red pepper flakes (optional)
- Salt and pepper to taste
- Olive oil for sautéing

Instructions:

Sauté Spinach:

- In a skillet, heat a little olive oil over medium heat.
- Add the chopped spinach and sauté until wilted. Remove from heat and put aside.

Prep Artichokes:

- Drain and slice the marinated artichoke hearts.

Blend Cheesy Mixture:

- Add the softened cream cheese, sour cream, mayonnaise, grated Parmesan cheese, shredded mozzarella cheese, minced garlic, red pepper flakes (if using), salt, and pepper in your Vitamix blender.

Blend Until Smooth:

- Blend on low speed, gradually increasing to high, until the mixture is smooth and thoroughly incorporated.

- Combine the sautéed spinach and chopped artichokes with the combined cheesy mixture in a mixing dish. Mix thoroughly.

- Transfer the mixture to a baking dish.

- Preheat your oven to 375°F (190°C).
- Bake the dip for approximately 20-25 minutes until the top is golden brown and the drop bubbles.

- Remove the dip from the oven and allow it to cool slightly before serving.

- Serve the Spinach and Artichoke Dip with dippers such as tortilla chips, sliced baguette, crackers, or veggie sticks.

- Savour the warm and cheesy tastes of this traditional dip.

This Spinach and Artichoke Dip is an excellent crowd-pleasing staple for events or just eating with friends and family. The combination of sautéed spinach, artichoke hearts, and a creamy, cheesy base offers a beautiful balance of tastes and textures that's impossible to resist.

Sun-Dried Tomato Pesto

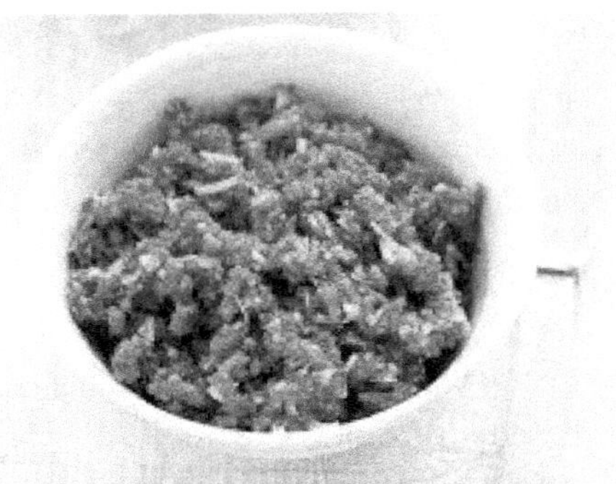

Elevate your meals with the robust tastes of this Sun-Dried Tomato Pesto. Bursting with the richness of sun-dried tomatoes, aromatic basil, and nutty pine nuts, this versatile spread offers a lovely flavour to pasta, sandwiches, or even dip.

Ingredients:

- 1 cup sun-dried tomatoes (dry-packed or oil-packed)
- 1 cup fresh basil leaves
- ½ cup grated Parmesan cheese
- 1/3 cup pine nuts, roasted
- Two cloves garlic, minced
- ½ cup extra-virgin olive oil
- Juice of 1 lemon
- Salt and pepper to taste

Soak Sun-Dried Tomatoes:

- If using dry-packed sun-dried tomatoes, soak them in boiling water for approximately 15 minutes to soften. If using oil-packed sun-dried tomatoes, rinse and pat them dry.

Toast Pine Nuts:

- In a dry pan over medium heat, toast the pine nuts until lightly brown and aromatic. Be careful to stir often to avoid burning.

Blend Ingredients:

- Add the soaked sun-dried tomatoes (drained if soaked), fresh basil leaves, grated Parmesan cheese, roasted pine nuts, minced garlic, and lemon juice in your Vitamix blender.

Blend Until Smooth:

- Blend on low speed, gradually increasing to high, until the mixture combines finely and forms a thick paste.

Drizzle in Olive Oil:

- Carefully trickle in the extra-virgin olive oil with the low-speed blender until the pesto reaches your desired consistency.

Taste and Adjust:

- Taste the pesto and season with salt and pepper as required. You may also modify the acidity by adding extra lemon juice if desired.

Serve and Store:

- Transfer the Sun-Dried Tomato Pesto to a jar or airtight container.

- Store in the refrigerator for up to a week, or freeze in little quantities for extended storage.

- Enjoy the pesto as a spaghetti sauce, sandwich spread, or dip for breadsticks or veggie crudités.

- Get creative by using this pesto in numerous recipes – from pasta and pizza to salads and wraps.

This Sun-Dried Tomato Pesto is a burst of flavour that adds a touch of elegance to your dishes. The sun-dried tomatoes add richness, while the mix of basil, pine nuts, and Parmesan cheese lends depth and texture to the blend. This pesto will complement your gourmet masterpieces, whether used as a sauce or spread.

Black Bean Dip

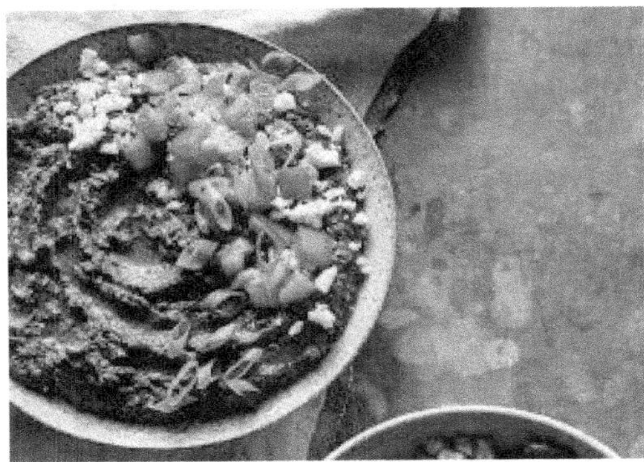

Savour the flavours of this spicy and protein-packed Black Bean Dip. With the earthiness of black beans, the zing of lime juice, and the warmth of spices, this dip is excellent for dipping tortilla chips and vegetable sticks or as a savoury complement to tacos and burritos.

Ingredients:

- Two cans (15 oz each) of black beans, drained and rinsed
- ¼ cup fresh cilantro, chopped
- Two cloves garlic, minced
- Juice of 2 limes
- One teaspoon of ground cumin
- ½ teaspoon chilli powder
- ¼ teaspoon cayenne pepper (adjust to taste)
- Salt and pepper to taste
- 2 tablespoons olive oil
- Optional toppings: chopped tomatoes, diced red onion, crumbled queso fresco or feta cheese

Instructions:

Blend Bean Mixture:

- Add the drained and rinsed black beans, chopped cilantro, minced garlic, lime juice, ground cumin, chilli powder, cayenne pepper, salt, and pepper in your Vitamix blender.

Blend Until Smooth:

- Blend on low speed, gradually increasing to high, until the mixture is smooth and creamy.

Drizzle in Olive Oil:

- With the blender running on low speed, carefully trickle in the olive oil to give richness and smoothness to the dip.

Adjust Seasonings:

- Taste the dip and adjust the spices to your satisfaction. Add extra lime juice, herbs, or salt as required.

Serve and Garnish:

- Transfer the Black Bean Dip to a serving dish.

Garnish and Customize:

- Customize the dip by garnishing it with chopped tomatoes, diced red onion, and crumbled queso fresco or feta cheese.

Pair with Dippers:

- Serve the dip with tortilla chips, carrot sticks, bell pepper slices, or any of your favourite dippers.

Enjoy the Zesty Flavors:

- Relish the zesty and spicy tones of this protein-rich dip.

This Black Bean Dip gives a flavour and a pleasing texture that's excellent for parties, gatherings, or even a fast snack. The mix of black beans and spicy spices makes a dip that's both substantial and tasty. Use it as a dip, spread, or even a filler for tacos and burritos to offer a wonderful twist to your meals.

Baba Ganoush

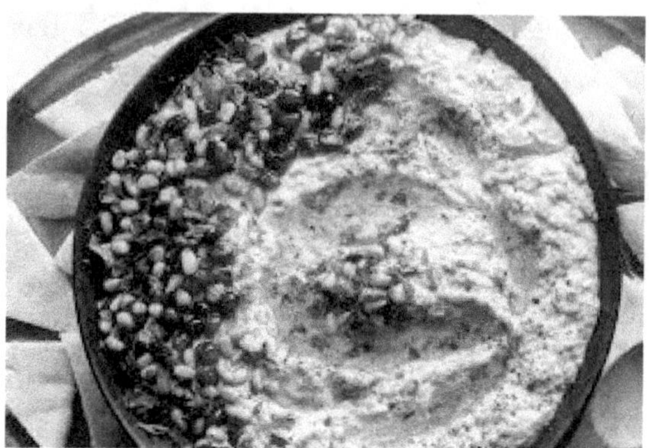

Delight in the smoky and creamy tastes of this classic Middle Eastern dip, Baba Ganoush. Made with roasted eggplant, tahini, and various spices, this dip is ideal for dipping pita bread, fresh veggies or as a spread in sandwiches and wraps.

Ingredients:

- Two medium eggplants
- ¼ cup tahini
- Three cloves garlic, minced
- Juice of 1 lemon
- 2 tablespoons extra-virgin olive oil, plus more for drizzling
- ½ teaspoon ground cumin
- Salt and pepper to taste
- Chopped fresh parsley for garnish
- Optional toppings: pomegranate seeds, roasted pine nuts, chopped fresh mint

Roast Eggplants:
- Preheat your oven to 400°F (200°C).
- Prick the eggplants with a fork and set them on a baking pan.
- Roast the eggplants in the oven for approximately 40-45 minutes or until the skin is browned and the meat is tender.

Cool and Peel:
- Once roasted, remove the eggplants from the oven and allow them to cool slightly.
- Peel off the burned skin and discard.

Blend Eggplant Mixture:
- Add roasted eggplant flesh, tahini, minced garlic, lemon juice, extra-virgin olive oil, ground cumin, salt, and pepper in your Vitamix blender.

Blend Until Smooth:
- Blend on low speed, gradually increasing to high, until the mixture is smooth and creamy.

Taste and Adjust:
- Taste the Baba Ganoush and adjust the spices by adding additional lemon juice, tahini, or salt as required.

Serve and Garnish:
- Transfer the Baba Ganoush to a serving dish.

Garnish and Customize:
- Garnish the dip with chopped fresh parsley.

- You may top with pomegranate seeds, toasted pine nuts, or chopped fresh mint for extra aesthetic appeal and taste.

Pair with Dippers:

- Serve the dip with pita bread, toasted pita chips, cucumber slices, or carrot sticks.

Enjoy the Smoky Creaminess:

- Relish the smokey and velvety texture of this traditional Middle Eastern dip.

Baba Ganoush delivers a unique and delectable combination of tastes guaranteed to satisfy your palette. The smokey undertones from the roasted eggplant, mixed with the nuttiness of tahini and the brightness of lemon juice, produce a dip that's both gratifying and unusual. Whether served as an appetizer or a snack, this dip will transport you to the bright tastes of the Middle East.

Spicy Salsa Verde

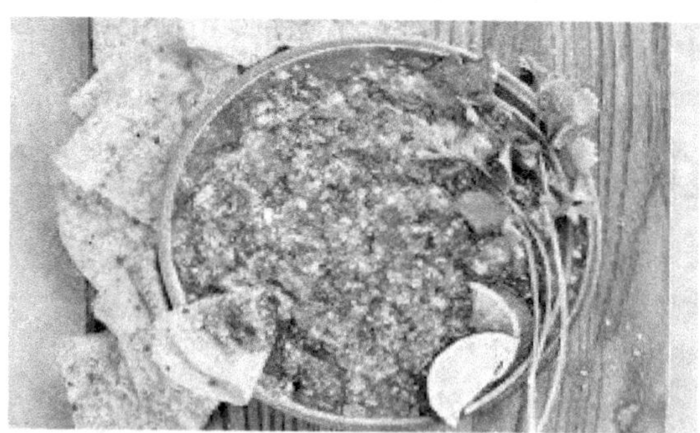

Embrace the spicy and colourful tastes of this Spicy Salsa Verde, a tangy green salsa excellent for dipping, topping, or adding spice to your favourite recipes. With the zing of tomatillos, the zest of jalapenos, and the freshness of cilantro, this salsa is guaranteed to improve your dishes.

Ingredients:

- Six tomatillos, husked and washed
- 2-3 jalapeño peppers (modify to taste)
- ½ onion, chopped
- Two cloves garlic, minced
- ¼ cup fresh cilantro leaves
- Juice of 2 limes
- Salt and pepper to taste

Instructions:

Char Tomatillos with Jalapenos:

- Preheat your broiler or grill on high heat.
- Place the tomatillos and jalapenos on a baking sheet or the grill grates.
- Char the tomatillos and jalapenos on both sides until they are blistered and slightly browned.

Blend Salsa Mixture:

- Add the charred tomatillos, charred jalapenos (stem and seeds removed for reduced heat), chopped onion, minced garlic, fresh cilantro leaves, lime juice, salt, and pepper in your Vitamix blender.

Blend to Desired Consistency:

- Blend on low speed, gradually increasing to high, until the salsa achieves your desired consistency. Leave it somewhat lumpy or mix till smooth.

Adjust Heat and Seasonings:

- Taste the salsa and adjust the heat by adding additional jalapenos if required.
- Season with extra salt and pepper if required.

Serve and Enjoy:

- Transfer the Spicy Salsa Verde to a serving dish.

Pair with Dippers:

- Serve the salsa with tortilla chips, tacos, grilled meats, or as a topping for enchiladas.

Savour the Zing:

- Revel in the zesty and spicy aromas of this bright salsa.

This Spicy Salsa Verde gives a rush of freshness and spice guaranteed to stimulate your taste senses. The charred tomatillos, jalapenos, and other tasty ingredients make an energetic and flexible salsa. This salsa is a must-have addition to your culinary arsenal, whether used for dipping, drizzling, or topping.

Whipped Feta with Herb Spread

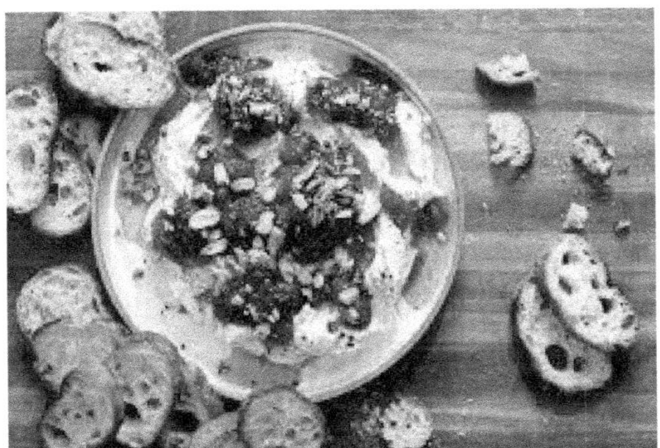

Indulge in the exquisite tastes of this Whipped Feta & Herb Spread, a creamy and tangy dip enhanced with the richness of feta cheese and the freshness of herbs. Perfect for spreading over crackers, crusty toast, or serving as a dip for veggies.

Ingredients:

- 8 ounces feta cheese, crumbled
- ¼ cup plain Greek yogurt
- Two tablespoons fresh chives chopped two tablespoons fresh dill, chopped two tablespoons fresh parsley, chopped one clove garlic, minced.
- Zest of 1 lemon
- Juice of ½ lemon
- Two tablespoons extra-virgin olive oil
- Salt and pepper to taste

Instructions:

Blend Feta Mixture:

- Add the crumbled feta cheese, plain Greek yogurt, chopped chives, chopped dill, chopped parsley, minced garlic, lemon zest, lemon juice, extra-virgin olive oil, salt, and pepper in your Vitamix blender.

Blend Until Creamy:

- Blend on low speed, gradually increasing to high, until the mixture is creamy and smooth.

Adjust Consistency:

- If the spread is too thick, add a splash of water or olive oil to obtain the correct consistency.

Taste and Adjust:

- Taste the spread and adjust the spices by adding additional lemon juice, salt, or herbs.

Serve and Garnish:

- Transfer the Whipped Feta and Herb Spread to a serving dish.

Garnish and Customize:

- Garnish the spread with fresh chopped herbs and a drizzle of olive oil for a touch of sophistication.

Pair with Dippers:

- Serve the spread with dippers such as crackers, toasted baguette slices, or veggie sticks.

Enjoy the Creaminess:

- Relish the creamy and tangy tastes of this delectable spread.

This Whipped Feta, and Herb Spread is a delicious blend of creamy feta cheese and the fragrant freshness of herbs. The balance of tastes and textures produces a refined and appealing spread. Whether served as an appetizer, party plate addition, or a simple snack, this spread is guaranteed to wow with its decadent flavour.

Curry Cashew Dip

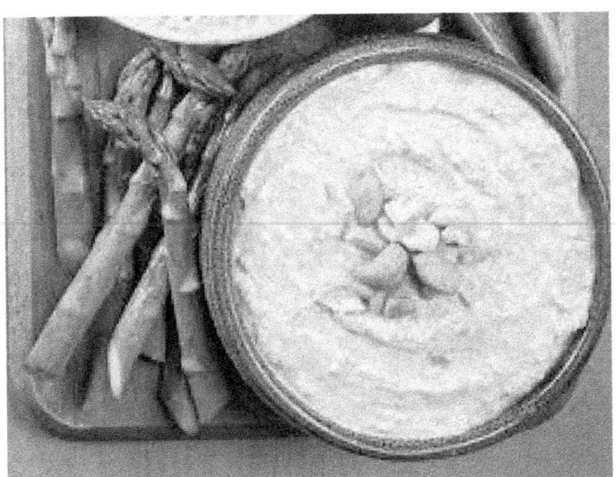

Experience the delicious blend of flavours in this Curry Cashew Dip. Combining the nutty richness of cashews with the warmth of curry spices, this dip is a unique and tasty alternative for dipping vegetables, pita bread, or as a spread on sandwiches.

Ingredients:

- 1 cup raw cashews, soaked and drained
- One tablespoon of curry powder
- One teaspoon of ground cumin

- ½ teaspoon ground turmeric
- ¼ teaspoon ground coriander
- ¼ teaspoon cayenne pepper (adjust to taste)
- Juice of 1 lemon
- Two cloves garlic, minced
- Two tablespoons extra-virgin olive oil
- ¼ cup water (or more for desired consistency)
- Salt and pepper to taste

Instructions:

Soak Cashews:

- Place the raw cashews in a dish and cover them with water. Let them soak for at least 2 hours, preferably overnight. Drain and rinse before using.

Blend Cashew Mixture:

- In your Vitamix blender, add the soaked and drained cashews, curry powder, powdered cumin, ground turmeric, ground coriander, cayenne pepper, lemon juice, chopped garlic, extra-virgin olive oil, water, salt, and pepper.

Blend Until Smooth:

- Blend on low speed, gradually increasing to high, until the mixture is smooth and creamy. Add extra water as required to attain the desired consistency.

Adjust Seasonings:

- Taste the Curry Cashew Dip and adjust the spices by adding additional curry powder, lemon juice, or salt to your satisfaction.

- Transfer the dip to a serving dish.

- Serve the dip with dippers such as carrot sticks, bell pepper slices, cucumber rounds, or warm pita bread.

- Revel in the perfect combination of nuts, cashews, and fragrant Thai spices.

This Curry Cashew Dip provides a delicious change from usual dips, filling your taste senses with a rush of warmth and nuttiness. The mix of spicy spices and creamy cashews makes a pleasant and fascinating dip. Whether consumed as a snack, appetizer, or sandwich spread, this dip is guaranteed to bring a bit of international flare to your meals.

Caramelized Onion Dip

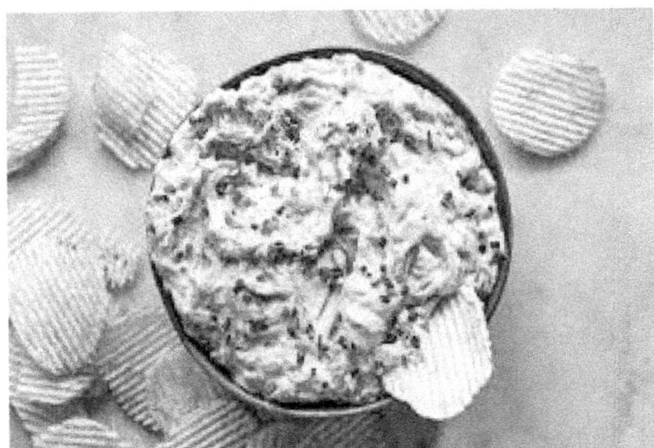

Indulge in the rich and sweet tastes of our Caramelized Onion Dip. Made with lusciously caramelized onions and accented by creamy sour cream and mayonnaise; this dip is excellent for combining with chips, crackers, or veggie sticks.

Ingredients:

- Two big onions, thinly sliced
- Two tablespoons butter
- One tablespoon of olive oil
- 1 cup sour cream
- ½ cup mayonnaise
- One teaspoon of Worcestershire sauce
- Salt and pepper to taste
- Chopped fresh chives for garnish

Instructions:

Caramelize Onions:

- Melt the butter and olive oil in a large pan over medium-low heat.
- Add the thinly sliced onions and heat, turning regularly, until they become golden brown and are caramelized. This should take 20-25 minutes. Be patient since prolonged simmering brings out the sweetness in the onions.

Cool Onions:

- Allow the caramelized onions to cool to room temperature.

Blend Dip Mixture:

- Add the cooled caramelized onions, sour cream, mayonnaise, Worcestershire sauce, salt, and pepper in your Vitamix blender.

- Blend on low speed, gradually increasing to high, until the mixture is smooth and thoroughly incorporated.

- Taste the Caramelized Onion Dip and adjust the spices as required by adding additional salt, pepper, or Worcestershire sauce.

- Transfer the dip to a serving dish.

- Garnish the dip with chopped fresh chives for an added layer of flavour and aesthetic appeal.

- Serve the dip with dippable potato chips, pretzels, crackers, or veggie sticks.

- Relish the sweetness of caramelized onions coupled with the creaminess of the dip.

This Caramelized Onion Dip lends a sense of refinement and sophistication to your snacking experience. The labour of love in caramelizing the onions is worth it, as it gives a depth of flavour that's tempting. Whether eaten at parties or for a peaceful night, this dip is guaranteed to be a crowd-pleaser with its luxurious and excellent taste.

CHAPTER FIVE

Acai and Superfood Bowls

Classic Acai Bowl

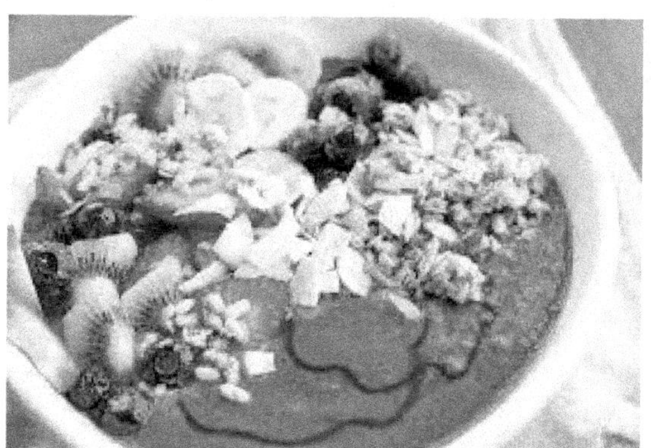

Indulge in the refreshing and nutritional deliciousness of a Classic Acai Bowl. Packed with antioxidants and topped with delectable toppings, this bowl is a fantastic way to start your day or enjoy as a fulfilling snack.

Ingredients:

- Two packets (approximately 3.5 ounces each) of frozen acai puree
- One ripe banana
- ¼ cup almond milk (or your chosen milk)
- Toppings: granola, sliced banana, berries (such as strawberries, blueberries, raspberries), honey or agave nectar, shredded coconut

Instructions:

Prep Acai Packets:

- Run the frozen acai packets under warm water for a few seconds to gently soften. Break them into little pieces for easy mixing.

Blend Acai Mixture:

- Add softened acai, ripe banana, and almond milk to your Vitamix blender.

Blend Until Smooth:

- Start mixing on low speed and gradually raise to high. Blend until the mixture is smooth and thick.

Adjust Consistency:

- If the mixture is too thick, add more almond milk to obtain your preferred consistency.

Prepare Toppings:

- Slice more bananas and collect your choice of fruit.

Assemble Acai Bowl:

- Pour the pureed acai mixture into a bowl.

Add Toppings:

- Arrange sliced bananas, berries, and granola in the acai mixture.

Drizzle with Sweetener:

- Drizzle honey or agave nectar over the toppings for a hint of sweetness.

Optional Coconut:

- Sprinkle shredded coconut over the top for more taste and texture.

Enjoy the Acai Bowl:

- Grab a spoon and appreciate your Classic Acai Bowl's colourful tastes and textures.

This Classic Acai Bowl is a delicious blend of creamy acai, naturally sweet banana, and various colourful toppings. It's aesthetically stunning and filled with essential nutrients to fuel your day. Customize the toppings to your taste and enjoy a tasty and healthful treat suitable for any time of day.

Tropical Acai Bowl

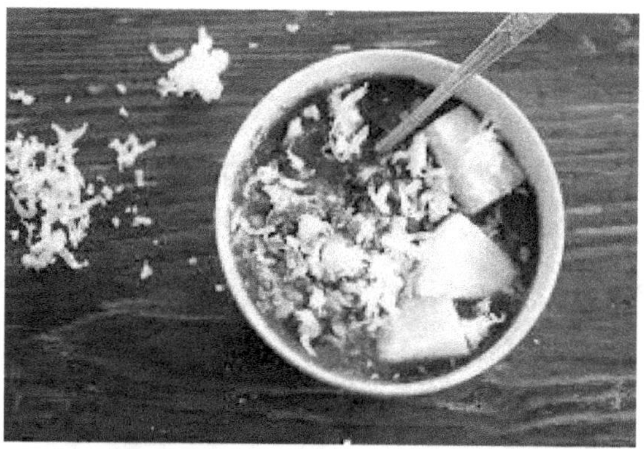

Transport yourself to a tropical paradise with the refreshing and vivid tastes of a Tropical Acai Bowl. Bursting with tropical fruits and acai deliciousness, this bowl is a great way to start your morning or enjoy a taste of sunshine any time.

- Two packets (approximately 3.5 ounces each) of frozen acai puree
- ½ cup frozen pineapple chunks
- ½ cup frozen mango chunks
- ½ cup coconut water or coconut milk
- Juice of 1 lime
- Toppings: sliced mango, sliced banana, kiwi slices, shredded coconut, chia seeds, chopped fresh mint

Instructions:

Prep Acai Packets:

- Run the frozen acai packets under warm water for a few seconds to gently soften. Break them into little pieces for easy mixing.

Blend Acai Mixture:

- Add softened acai, pineapple, mango, coconut water (or coconut milk), and lime juice in your Vitamix blender.

Blend Until Smooth:

- Start mixing on low speed and gradually raise to high. Blend until the mixture is smooth and creamy.

Adjust Consistency:

- Add more coconut water or coconut milk to obtain your preferred consistency if the mixture is too thick.

Prepare Toppings:

- Slice mango, banana, and kiwi. Chop fresh mint leaves.

Assemble Acai Bowl:

- Pour the pureed acai mixture into a bowl.

- Arrange the sliced mango, banana, and kiwi on top of the acai mixture.

- Sprinkle shredded coconut and chia seeds over the toppings for added taste and nutrition.

- Garnish with chopped fresh mint leaves for a blast of freshness.

- Dive into the tropical paradise of flavours with each mouthful of your Tropical Acai Bowl.

This Tropical Acai Bowl delivers the tastes of the tropics directly to your bowl. The mix of acai, pineapple, mango, and coconut makes a refreshing and exhilarating blend that's excellent for a warm day or when you want to taste exotic. Customize the toppings to your preference and enjoy this bowl's bright and tasty experience.

Mixed Berry Acai Bowl

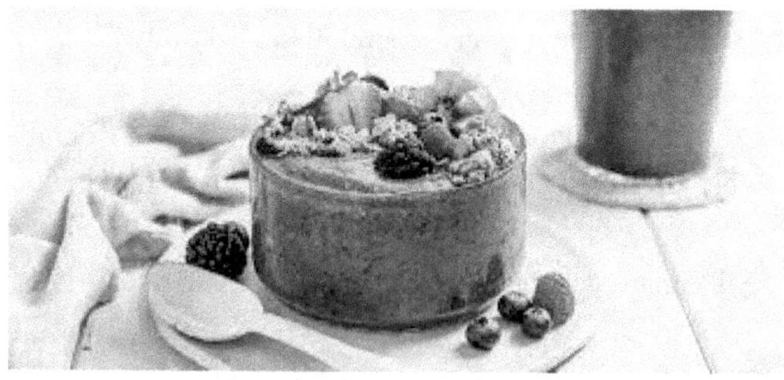

Indulge in the colourful and antioxidant-rich tastes of a Mixed Berry Acai Bowl. Combining the richness of acai with a mixture of berries, this bowl gives a rush of sweetness and nutrition that's great for a healthful breakfast or snack.

- Two packets (approximately 3.5 ounces each) of frozen acai puree
- ½ cup mixed berries (strawberries, blueberries, raspberries)
- ¼ cup plain Greek yogurt
- ¼ cup almond milk (or your chosen milk)
- One tablespoon of honey or maple syrup
- Toppings: mixed berries, granola, sliced banana, chopped nuts (such as almonds or walnuts), a sprinkle of honey

- Run the frozen acai packets under warm water for a few seconds to gently soften. Break them into little pieces for easy mixing.

- Add the softened acai, mixed berries, plain Greek yogurt, almond milk, and honey (or maple syrup) in your Vitamix blender.

- Start mixing on low speed and gradually raise to high. Blend until the mixture is smooth and creamy.

- If the mixture is too thick, add more almond milk to obtain your preferred consistency.

- Pour the pureed acai mixture into a bowl.

- Arrange a selection of mixed berries, granola, sliced banana, and chopped almonds on top of the acai mixture.

- Drizzle a little honey over the toppings for an added touch of sweetness.

- Dive into the delightful and colourful world of your Mixed Berry Acai Bowl.

This Mixed Berry Acai Bowl blends the health of acai with the natural sweetness of mixed berries. The Greek yogurt gives smoothness and a protein boost, while the diversity of toppings adds texture and taste to each mouthful. Customize the toppings to your desire and enjoy a healthy and enjoyable bowl that's as beautiful to the eyes as it is to the taste sensations.

Green Acai Bowl

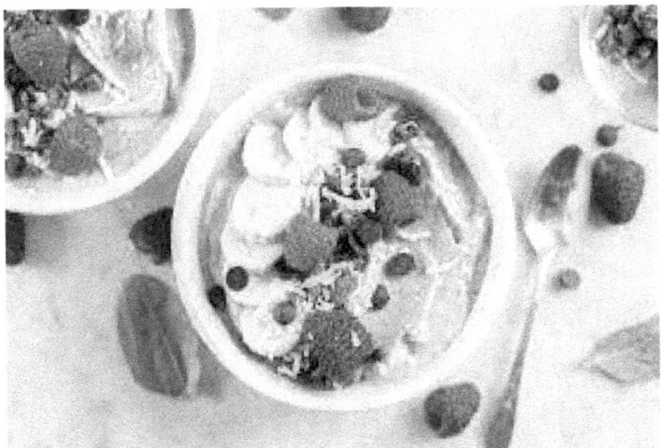

Embrace the nutritious and colourful tastes of a Green Acai Bowl. Packed with nutrients and lush greens, this bowl gives your day a refreshing and energetic start.

Ingredients:

- Two packets (approximately 3.5 ounces each) of frozen acai puree
- 1 cup fresh spinach leaves
- ½ cup fresh kale leaves, stems removed
- One ripe banana
- ½ cup almond milk (or your chosen milk)
- One teaspoon spirulina or chlorella powder (optional, for extra green colour and nutrients)
- Toppings: sliced kiwi, sliced banana, chia seeds, pumpkin seeds, hemp seeds

Prep Acai Packets:

- Run the frozen acai packets under warm water for a few seconds to gently soften. Break them into little pieces for easy mixing.

Blend Acai Mixture:

- Add softened acai, spinach, kale, ripe banana, almond milk, spirulina, or chlorella powder in your Vitamix blender.

Blend Until Smooth:

- Start mixing on low speed and gradually raise to high. Blend until the mixture is smooth and brilliant green.

Adjust Consistency:

- If the mixture is too thick, add more almond milk to obtain your preferred consistency.

Assemble Acai Bowl:

- Pour the pureed acai mixture into a bowl.

Add Toppings:

- Arrange sliced kiwi, banana, chia, pumpkin, and hemp seeds on top of the acai mixture.

Enjoy the Green Goodness:

- Delight in the refreshing and nutrient-packed tastes of your Green Acai Bowl.

This Green Acai Bowl delivers a nutritional combination of acai, leafy greens, and refreshing and invigorating superfoods. Including spirulina or chlorella powder increases the brilliant green colour while offering extra nutrients. Customize the toppings to your desire and enjoy a bowl that tastes delicious and gives you a healthful start to your day.

Chocolate Acai Bowl

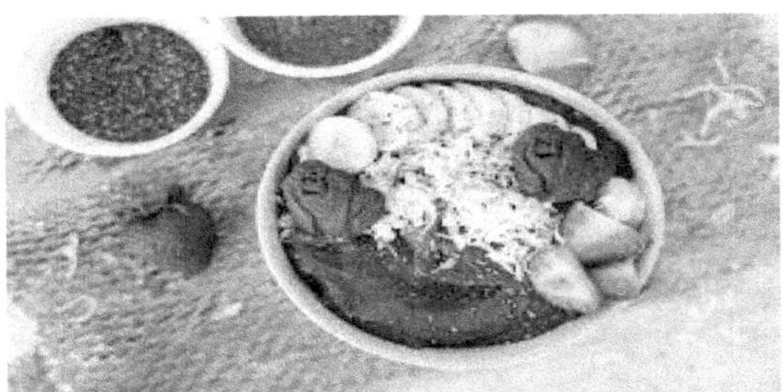

Indulge in the luscious and rich tastes of a Chocolate Acai Bowl. Combining the health of acai with the tempting flavour of chocolate, this bowl is a beautiful treat that's excellent for fulfilling your sweet cravings.

Ingredients:

- Two packets (approximately 3.5 ounces each) of frozen acai puree
- 1 ripe banana
- Two teaspoons of cacao powder
- ½ cup almond milk (or your chosen milk)
- One tablespoon of nut butter (such as almond or peanut butter)
- Toppings: cacao nibs, chopped nuts (such as almonds or hazelnuts), sliced banana, a drizzle of nut butter

Instructions:

Prep Acai Packets:

- Run the frozen acai packets under warm water for a few seconds to gently soften. Break them into little pieces for easy mixing.

Blend Acai Mixture:

- Add softened acai, ripe banana, cacao powder, almond milk, and nut butter to your Vitamix blender.

Blend Until Smooth:

- Start mixing on low speed and gradually raise to high. Blend until the mixture is smooth and chocolaty.

Adjust Consistency:

- If the mixture is too thick, add more almond milk to obtain your preferred consistency.

Assemble Acai Bowl:

- Pour the pureed acai mixture into a bowl.

Add Toppings:

- Sprinkle cacao nibs, chopped almonds, and sliced banana on the chocolate acai mixture.

Drizzle with Nut Butter:

- Drizzle a little nut butter over the toppings for an added layer of flavour.

Savour the Chocolate Bliss:

- Indulge in the rich and beautiful tastes of your Chocolate Acai Bowl.

This Chocolate Acai Bowl provides a new spin on typical acai bowls, blending the lusciousness of chocolate with the nutritious advantages of acai. The combination of cacao powder and nut butter offers a delightful treat that's excellent for dessert or anytime you're seeking something sweet and chocolatey. Customize the toppings to your preference and enjoy a delicious guilt-free and delicious bowl of chocolate.

Berry Protein Acai Bowl

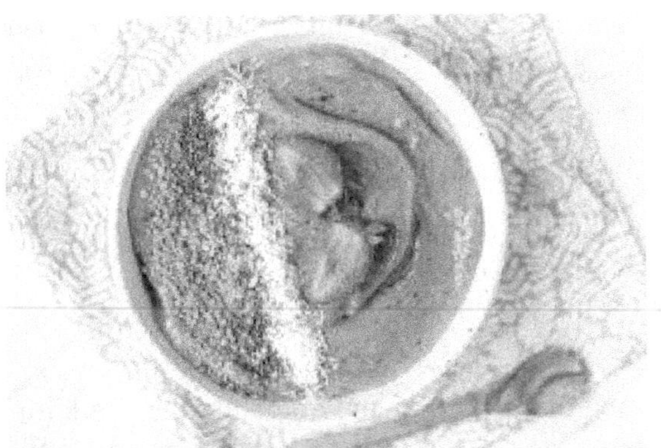

Elevate your acai bowl experience with a blast of protein and the benefits of mixed berries. This Berry Protein Acai Bowl is tasty and a terrific way to power your day with critical nutrients.

Ingredients:

- Two packets (approximately 3.5 ounces each) of frozen acai puree
- ½ cup mixed berries (strawberries, blueberries, raspberries)
- One scoop of your preferred protein powder (such as plant-based or whey)
- ¼ cup plain Greek yogurt

- ¼ cup almond milk (or your chosen milk)
- Toppings: granola, mixed berries, sliced banana, chopped nuts (such as almonds or walnuts), a drizzle of honey

Instructions:

Prep Acai Packets:

- Run the frozen acai packets under warm water for a few seconds to gently soften. Break them into little pieces for easy mixing.

Blend Acai Mixture:

- Add the softened acai, mixed berries, protein powder, plain Greek yogurt, and almond milk in your Vitamix blender.

Blend Until Smooth:

- Start mixing on low speed and gradually raise to high. Blend until the mixture is smooth and fully incorporated.

Adjust Consistency:

- If the mixture is too thick, add more almond milk to obtain your preferred consistency.

Assemble Acai Bowl:

- Pour the pureed acai mixture into a bowl.

Add Toppings:

- Sprinkle granola, mixed berries, sliced banana, and chopped almonds on top of the protein-packed acai combination.

Drizzle with Honey:

- Drizzle some honey over the toppings for a hint of natural sweetness.

Enjoy the Protein Boost:

- Delight in your Berry Protein Acai Bowl's healthy tastes and protein-rich richness.

This Berry Protein Acai Bowl is a terrific alternative for people wanting a mix of protein, vitamins, and antioxidants in their diet. Combining acai, mixed berries, and protein powder delivers a delightful and healthy solution to fuel your active lifestyle. Customize the toppings to your choice and enjoy a bowl that keeps you full and energetic throughout the day.

Acai Peanut Butter Bowl

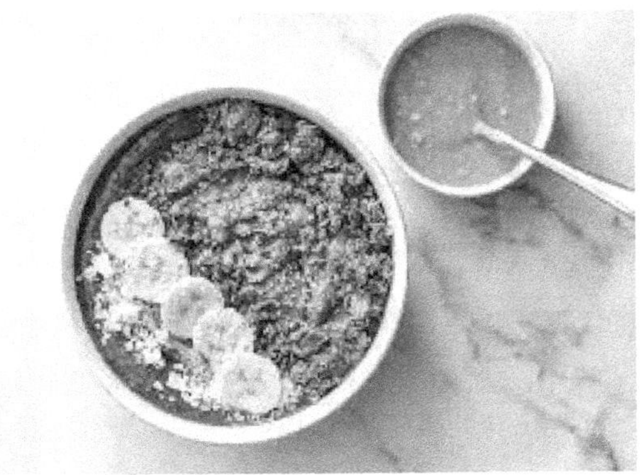

Satisfy your needs for both sweet and savoury with the delectable blend of acai and peanut butter in this Acai Peanut Butter Bowl. Creamy and rich, this bowl is a beautiful treat that's excellent for breakfast or a fulfilling snack.

Ingredients:

- Two packets (approximately 3.5 ounces each) of frozen acai puree
- 1 ripe banana
- 2 tbsp peanut butter
- ½ cup almond milk (or your chosen milk)
- Toppings: sliced banana, chopped peanuts, dab of peanut butter, granola, cacao nibs (optional)

Instructions:

Prep Acai Packets:

- Run the frozen acai packets under warm water for a few seconds to gently soften. Break them into little pieces for easy mixing.

Blend Acai Mixture:

- Add softened acai, ripe banana, peanut butter, and almond milk in your Vitamix blender.

Blend Until Smooth:

- Start mixing on low speed and gradually raise to high. Blend until the mixture is smooth and creamy.

Adjust Consistency:

- If the mixture is too thick, add more almond milk to obtain your preferred consistency.

Assemble Acai Bowl:

- Pour the pureed acai mixture into a bowl.

Add Toppings:

- Arrange sliced banana, chopped peanuts, and granola in the peanut butter-infused acai mixture.

Drizzle with Peanut Butter:

- Drizzle a large quantity of peanut butter over the toppings for an added layer of nutty flavour.

Optional Cacao Nibs:

- For a bit of chocolaty crunch, sprinkle cacao nibs over the bowl.

Enjoy the Peanutty Goodness:

- Dive into the beautiful and fulfilling tastes of your Acai Peanut Butter Bowl.

This Acai Peanut Butter Bowl uniquely combines rich acai, creamy peanut butter, and a kaleidoscope of delightful toppings. The mix of tastes and textures provides a delicate balance between sweet and savoury, making it an enjoyable but healthful meal. Customize the toppings to your choice and enjoy a soothing and energetic bowl.

Berry Matcha Acai Bowl

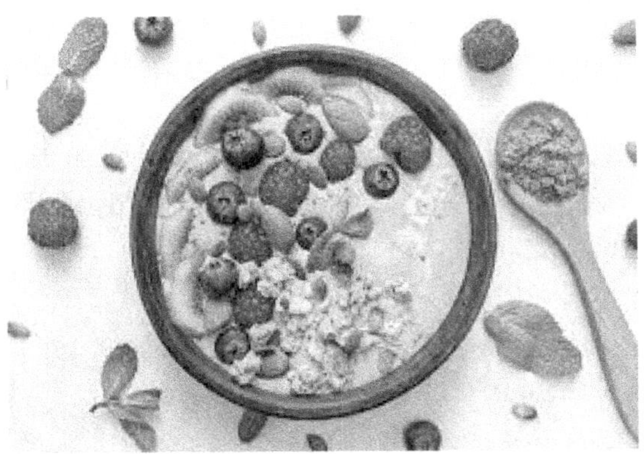

Experience the refreshing and antioxidant-packed richness of a Berry Matcha Acai Bowl. Combining the vivid aromas of berries with the distinct fragrance of matcha green tea, this bowl is a pleasant way to start your day on a healthy note.

Ingredients:

- Two packets (approximately 3.5 ounces each) of frozen acai puree
- ½ cup mixed berries (strawberries, blueberries, raspberries)
- 1 teaspoon matcha green tea powder
- ½ cup coconut water or almond milk
- Juice of ½ lemon
- Toppings: matcha granola, mixed berries, sliced banana, a sprinkle of matcha powder

Instructions:

Prep Acai Packets:

- Run the frozen acai packets under warm water for a few seconds to gently soften. Break them into little pieces for easy mixing.

Blend Acai Mixture:

- Add softened acai, mixed berries, matcha green tea powder, coconut water (or almond milk), and lemon juice in your Vitamix blender.

Blend Until Smooth:

- Start mixing on low speed and gradually raise to high. Blend until the mixture is smooth and vivid.

Adjust Consistency:

- If the mixture is too thick, add extra coconut water or almond milk to obtain your preferred consistency.

Assemble Acai Bowl:

- Pour the pureed acai mixture into a bowl.

Add Toppings:

- Sprinkle matcha granola, mixed berries, and sliced banana on top of the matcha-infused acai mixture.

Sprinkle with Matcha Powder:

- For a blast of matcha flavour and colour, sprinkle a dab of matcha powder over the toppings.

Enjoy the Matcha Bliss:

- Revel in the exhilarating and reviving tastes of your Berry Matcha Acai Bowl.

This Berry Matcha Acai Bowl delivers a mix of antioxidant-rich berries with the bright flavour of matcha green tea. The matcha provides a distinctive taste and a modest energy boost. Customize the toppings to your preference and enjoy a bowl that's healthful and a great gourmet experience.

CHAPTER SIX

Flavorful Sauces & Dressings

Creamy Caesar Dressing

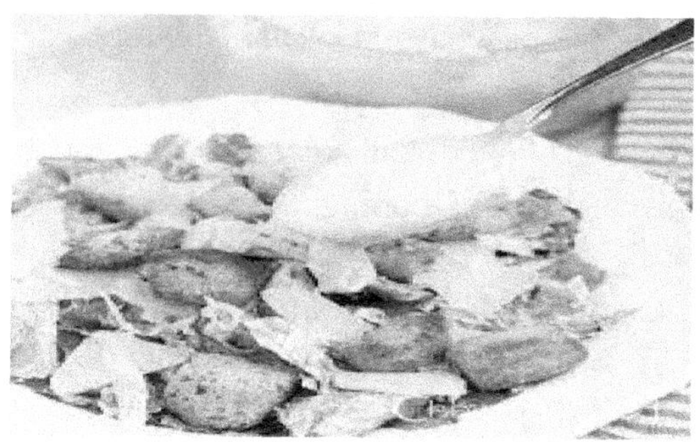

Indulge in the traditional and creamy tastes of homemade Caesar dressing with this easy-to-make recipe. Perfect for spreading over fresh Romaine lettuce or as a veggie dipping sauce.

Ingredients:

- ½ cup mayonnaise
- ¼ cup grated Parmesan cheese two teaspoons lemon juice
- One tablespoon of Dijon mustard
- Two cloves garlic, minced
- One teaspoon anchovy paste (optional)
- ¼ teaspoon black pepper
- Salt to taste

- ¼ cup olive oil

- Add mayonnaise, grated Parmesan cheese, lemon juice, Dijon mustard, chopped garlic, anchovy paste (if using), black pepper, and a touch of salt in your Vitamix blender.

- Start mixing on low speed and gradually raise to high. Blend until the sauce is smooth and all the components are properly blended.

- With the blender running on medium speed, carefully dribble in the olive oil until the dressing is creamy and emulsified.

- Taste the dressing and adjust the seasoning by adding additional salt, pepper, or lemon juice if desired.

- Transfer the creamy Caesar dressing to a glass jar or airtight container.

- Store the dressing in the refrigerator for approximately one week. Shake or mix thoroughly before each usage.

- Drizzle the Creamy Caesar Dressing over your favourite salads or use it as a dip for crudités. Enjoy the rich and traditional tastes!

Whether you're a lover of classic Caesar salads or searching for a flexible dressing for other meals, our Creamy Caesar Dressing provides the ideal blend of acidic, creamy, and umami tastes to your culinary creations.

Tangy Balsamic Vinaigrette

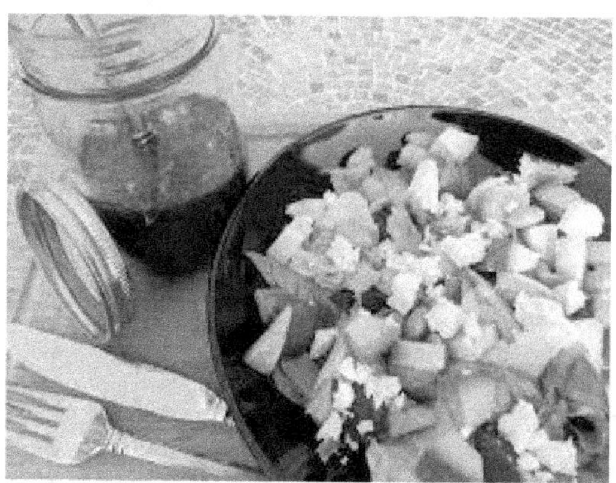

Elevate your salads with the beautiful blend of tanginess and sweetness in this handcrafted Balsamic Vinaigrette. Whip it up fast in your Vitamix blender for a dressing that compliments a range of greens and vegetables.

Ingredients:

- ¼ cup balsamic vinegar
- ½ cup extra-virgin olive oil
- One tablespoon of Dijon mustard
- One tablespoon honey
- One small shallot, minced

- Salt and black pepper to taste

- Add balsamic vinegar, extra-virgin olive oil, Dijon mustard, honey, chopped shallot, and a touch of salt and black pepper in your Vitamix blender.

- Start mixing on low speed and gradually raise to high. Blend until the ingredients are entirely emulsified and the dressing is smooth.

- Taste the dressing and adjust the seasoning by adding extra salt, pepper, or honey to your desire.

- Pour the tart Balsamic Vinaigrette into a glass jar or airtight container.

- Store the dressing in the refrigerator for up to 2 weeks. Shake thoroughly before each use.

- Drizzle the Tangy Balsamic Vinaigrette over your favourite salads for a blast of flavour. It also works excellent as a marinade for grilled vegetables and meats.

This Tangy Balsamic Vinaigrette has the ideal combination of acidity from the balsamic vinegar and sweetness from the honey, producing a versatile dressing that's fantastic for salads and more. Customize the ingredients to your liking and enjoy the delightful blend of tastes with every mouthful.

Spicy Sriracha Mayo

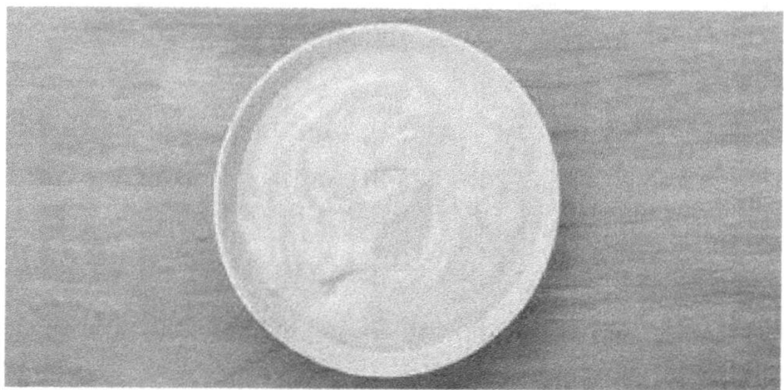

Add spice and flavour to your foods with our homemade Spicy Sriracha Mayo. Perfect as a dipping sauce, sandwich spread, or drizzle for a hint of spice.

Ingredients:

- ½ cup mayonnaise
- Two tablespoons Sriracha sauce (modify to taste)
- One tablespoon of lime juice
- One clove of garlic, minced
- One teaspoon honey
- Salt to taste

Blend Ingredients:
- Add mayonnaise, Sriracha sauce, lime juice, chopped garlic, honey, and a touch of salt in your Vitamix blender.

Blend Until Smooth:
- Start mixing on low speed and gradually raise to high. Blend until all the ingredients are thoroughly blended and the sauce smooths.

Taste and Adjust:
- Taste the Spicy Sriracha Mayo and adjust the flavour by adding additional Sriracha for increased heat, lime juice for tanginess, or honey for sweetness.

Transfer and Store:
- Transfer the sauce to a squeeze bottle or airtight container.

Refrigerate:
- Store the Spicy Sriracha Mayo in the refrigerator for approximately one week.

Serve and Enjoy:
- Use the sauce as a dip for fries, chicken tenders, veggies, a spread for burgers or sandwiches, or a drizzle over tacos. Enjoy the zesty and spicy tastes!

This Spicy Sriracha Mayo combines the robust tastes of Sriracha and the creamy richness of mayonnaise. Adjust the spiciness to your liking and use it to give an exciting kick to your favourite foods.

Fresh Pesto Sauce

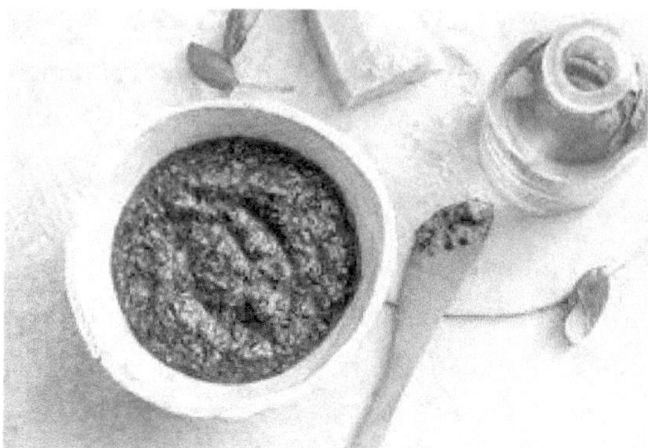

Elevate your pasta, sandwiches, and more with the rich and fragrant aromas of handmade Fresh Pesto Sauce. Whip up this traditional sauce using your Vitamix blender for a blast of basil flavour.

Ingredients:

- 2 cups fresh basil leaves, packed
- ½ cup grated Parmesan cheese
- ½ cup pine nuts or walnuts
- Three cloves garlic peeled
- ½ cup extra-virgin olive oil
- Salt and black pepper to taste

Instructions:

Blend Ingredients:

- Add fresh basil leaves, grated Parmesan cheese, pine nuts (or walnuts), peeled garlic cloves, and a sprinkling of salt and black pepper in your Vitamix blender.

Blend Until Smooth:

- Start mixing on low speed and gradually raise to high. Blend until the mixture is finely chopped.

Add Olive Oil:

- With the blender running on medium speed, carefully pour the extra-virgin olive oil until the sauce is smooth and thoroughly blended.

Taste and Adjust:

- Taste the Fresh Pesto Sauce and adjust the flavour by adding extra salt, pepper, or cheese as required.

Transfer and Store:

- Transfer the sauce to a glass jar or airtight container.

Refrigerate:

- Store the Fresh Pesto Sauce in the refrigerator for up to 1 week. To keep its brilliant green colour, spray a little olive oil coating on top before sealing.

Serve and Enjoy:

- Toss the Fresh Pesto Sauce with your favourite cooked pasta, spread it over sandwiches, use it as a marinade, or combine it into dips. Savour the fragrant and savoury essence!

This Fresh Pesto Sauce brings together the freshness of basil, the richness of Parmesan, and the nutty depth of pine nuts. Customize the ingredients and proportions to meet your taste preferences, and enjoy a flexible sauce that provides a rush of flavour to your gourmet masterpieces.

Zesty Avocado Lime Dressing

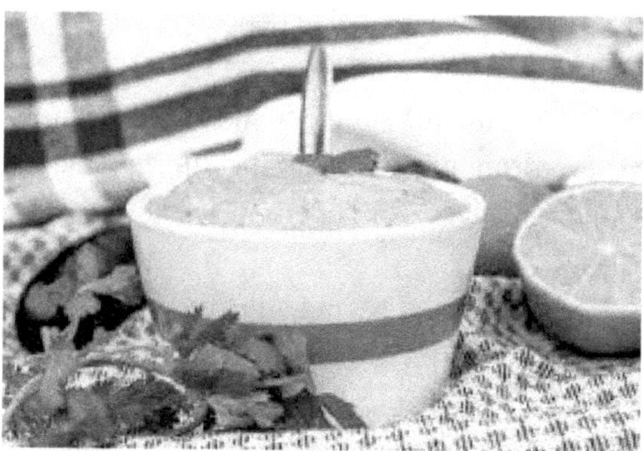

Experience the creamy deliciousness of avocado paired with the zesty tang of lime in this delectable Zesty Avocado Lime Dressing. Drizzle it over salads or grain bowls, or use it as a dip for a refreshing and savoury variation.

Ingredients:

- One ripe avocado, pitted and peeled
- Juice of 2 limes
- ¼ cup fresh cilantro leaves
- One clove garlic
- ¼ cup plain Greek yogurt
- Two tablespoons water
- Salt and black pepper to taste

Blend Ingredients:

- Add the ripe avocado, lime juice, fresh cilantro leaves, peeled garlic clove, plain Greek yogurt, and water in your Vitamix blender.

Blend Until Creamy:

- Start mixing on low speed and gradually raise to high. Blend until the mixture is smooth and creamy.

Adjust Consistency:

- Add more water to obtain your preferred consistency if the dressing is too thick.

Season and Taste:

- Add salt and a dash of black pepper to the dressing. Blend briefly to integrate.

Transfer and Store:

- Transfer the Zesty Avocado Lime Dressing to a glass jar or airtight container.

Refrigerate:

- Store the dressing in the refrigerator for up to 3 days. The avocado may cause minor browning, so use it reasonably quickly for the best colour.

Serve and Enjoy:

- Drizzle the Zesty Avocado Lime Dressing over salads, grain bowls, and tacos, or use it as a dip for veggies. Revel in the creamy avocado and zesty lime blend!

This Zesty Avocado Lime Dressing combines the smoothness of avocado and the zesty brightness of lime. Customize the ingredients and alter the tanginess to your taste choice. Enjoy a dressing that's not only tasty but also provides a beautiful splash of colour to your food.

Sesame Ginger Dressing

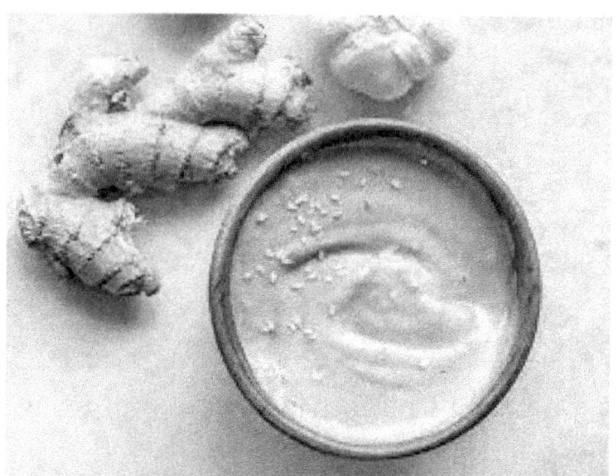

This delectable Sesame Ginger Dressing adds an Asian-inspired touch to your salads and meals. Bursting with the fragrant mix of sesame and ginger, this dressing is a versatile addition to your culinary arsenal.

Ingredients:

- ¼ cup sesame oil
- ¼ cup rice vinegar
- Two teaspoons of soy sauce
- One tablespoon of fresh ginger, peeled and grated
- One clove of garlic, minced
- One tablespoon of honey or maple syrup
- One teaspoon of sesame seeds
- Pinch of red pepper flakes (optional)

- Salt and black pepper to taste

Instructions:

Blend Ingredients:
- In your Vitamix blender, add sesame oil, rice vinegar, soy sauce, grated fresh ginger, minced garlic, honey (or maple syrup), sesame seeds, and a dash of red pepper flakes if needed.

Blend Until Combined:
- Start mixing on low speed and gradually raise to high. Blend until all the ingredients are properly incorporated.

Adjust Flavor:
- Taste the Sesame Ginger Dressing and adjust the flavour by adding salt, black pepper, or more sugar if needed.

Transfer and Store:
- Transfer the dressing to a glass jar or airtight container.

Refrigerate:
- Store the Sesame Ginger Dressing in the refrigerator for up to 1 week. Shake thoroughly before each use.

Serve and Enjoy:
- Drizzle the Sesame Ginger Dressing over salads, noodle meals, grilled veggies, or use it as a marinade for meats. Revel in the fragrant and savoury tastes!

This Sesame Ginger Dressing delivers a combination of nutty sesame and spicy ginger, producing a harmonic blend that's both flexible and tasty. Adjust the number of ingredients to suit your taste preferences and enjoy a dressing that may improve a wide variety of foods.

Creamy Tahini Dressing

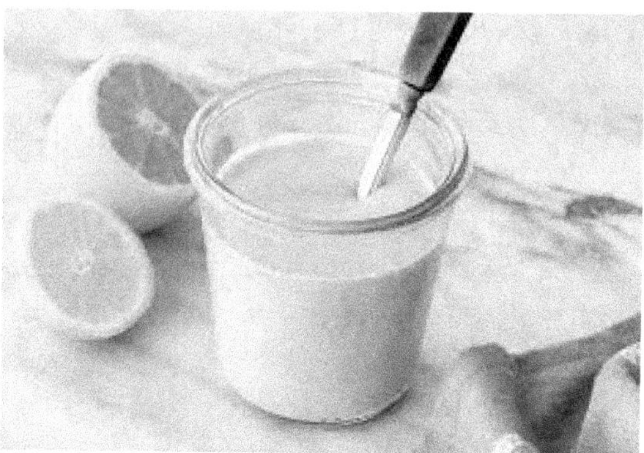

Experience the nutty richness of tahini paired with the acidic brightness of lemon juice in this fabulous Creamy Tahini Dressing. This dressing is versatile and savoury for salads, grain bowls, and more.

Ingredients:

- ¼ cup tahini
- Two teaspoons of lemon juice
- Two cloves garlic, minced
- Two tablespoons water
- Two tablespoons extra-virgin olive oil
- Salt and black pepper to taste
- **Optional:** chopped fresh herbs (such as parsley or dill)

Instructions:

Blend Ingredients:

- Add tahini, lemon juice, minced garlic, water, and extra-virgin olive oil in your Vitamix blender.

Blend Until Smooth:

- Start mixing on low speed and gradually raise to high. Blend till the mixture is creamy and fully incorporated.

Adjust Consistency:

- Add more water to obtain your preferred consistency if the dressing is too thick.

Season and Taste:

- Add salt and a dash of black pepper to the dressing. Blend briefly to integrate.

Optional Herbs:

- If desired, incorporate chopped fresh herbs like parsley or dill to improve the taste.

Transfer and Store:

- Transfer the Creamy Tahini Dressing to a glass jar or airtight container.

Refrigerate:

- Store the dressing in the refrigerator for up to 1 week. Stir or shake thoroughly before each use.

Serve and Enjoy:

- Drizzle the Creamy Tahini Dressing over salads, roasted veggies, or falafel, or use it as a dip for pita bread. Relish the silky and nutty tones!

This Creamy Tahini Dressing has a velvety texture and the unique flavour of tahini. Adjust the number of components to create your preferred taste profile. Enjoy a dressing that adds depth and creaminess to a variety of foods.

Cilantro Lime Dressing

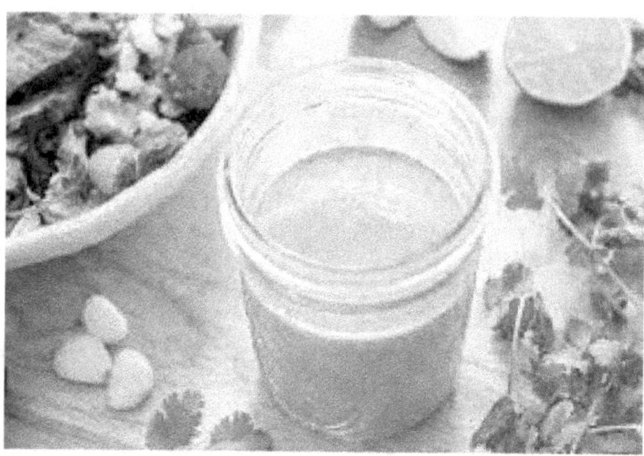

Elevate your meals with the vivid and spicy tastes of Cilantro Lime Dressing. Bursting with the freshness of cilantro and the sharpness of lime, this dressing is a versatile complement to salads, tacos, and more.

Ingredients:

- 1 cup fresh cilantro leaves and stems, packed
- Juice of 2 limes
- ¼ cup plain Greek yogurt
- One clove garlic
- One tablespoon of honey or maple syrup
- ¼ cup extra-virgin olive oil
- Salt and black pepper to taste

Blend Ingredients:

- Add fresh cilantro leaves and stems, lime juice, plain Greek yogurt, peeled garlic clove, honey (or maple syrup), and a sprinkling of salt and black pepper in your Vitamix blender.

Blend Until Smooth:

- Start mixing on low speed and gradually raise to high. Blend until the mixture is smooth and vivid.

Adjust Consistency:

- If the dressing is too thick, add more lime juice or water to obtain your preferred consistency.

Taste and Adjust:

- Taste the Cilantro Lime Dressing and adjust the flavour by adding additional salt, pepper, or sugar if needed.

Add Olive Oil:

- Carefully dribble in the extra-virgin olive oil with the blender running on medium speed until the dressing is thoroughly blended.

Transfer and Store:

- Transfer the dressing to a glass jar or airtight container.

Refrigerate:

- Store the Cilantro Lime Dressing in the refrigerator for up to 1 week. Stir thoroughly before each usage.

Serve and Enjoy:

- Drizzle the Cilantro Lime Dressing over salads, grilled chicken, or tacos, or use it as a dip for chips. Savour the tangy and herbaceous tastes!

This Cilantro Lime Dressing mixes the brightness of lime with the fragrant flavour of cilantro, producing a refreshing and adaptable dressing. Customize the ingredients and proportions to fit your taste preferences, and enjoy a sauce that adds a burst of flavour to your food.

Honey Mustard Sauce

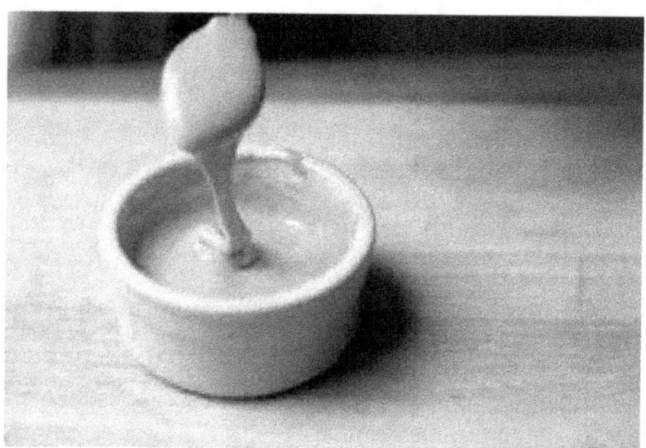

Indulge in the right combination of sweet and tangy with our homemade Honey Mustard Sauce. Drizzle it over salads and use it as a dipping sauce or a delicious marinade for your favourite foods.

Ingredients:

- ¼ cup Dijon mustard
- Two tablespoons honey
- Two tablespoons mayonnaise
- One tablespoon of apple cider vinegar
- ½ teaspoon paprika
- Salt and black pepper to taste

Instructions:

Blend Ingredients:

- Add Dijon mustard, honey, mayonnaise, apple cider vinegar, paprika, salt, and a dash of black pepper in your Vitamix blender.

Blend Until Smooth:

- Start mixing on low speed and gradually raise to high. Blend until the ingredients are fully incorporated, and the sauce is smooth.

Adjust Flavor:

- Taste the Honey Mustard Sauce and adjust the flavour by adding more honey for sweetness, mustard for tanginess, or salt & pepper.

Transfer and Store:

- Transfer the sauce to a glass jar or airtight container.

Refrigerate:

- Store the Honey Mustard Sauce in the refrigerator for up to 2 weeks. Stir thoroughly before each usage.

Serve and Enjoy:

- Drizzle the Honey Mustard Sauce over salads, use it as a dipping sauce for chicken tenders or pretzels, or use it as a grilled marinade. Enjoy the pleasant and balanced tastes!

This Honey Mustard Sauce mixes the robust tastes of Dijon mustard with the sweetness of honey. Customize the proportions to reach your ideal balance of sweet and tart. Enjoy a versatile sauce that may improve a range of foods.

CHAPTER SEVEN

Nutritious Main Dishes

Creamy Broccoli and Spinach Soup

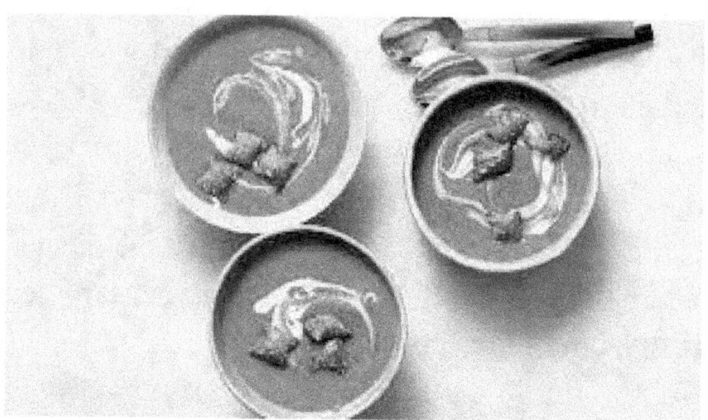

Indulge in the healthy pleasure of a Creamy Broccoli and Spinach Soup. This warm soup is rich with vitamins and taste, making it a fantastic option for a balanced supper.

Ingredients:

- 2 cups broccoli florets, cooked
- 2 cups fresh spinach leaves
- One small onion, chopped
- Two cloves garlic, minced
- 3 cups vegetable broth
- 1 cup unsweetened almond milk (or other plant-based milk)
- Two tablespoons of olive oil
- Salt and black pepper to taste

- Optional toppings: grated Parmesan, croutons, or a sprinkling of olive oil

Instructions:

Sauté Onion and Garlic:

- In a saucepan, heat the olive oil over medium heat. Add chopped onion and minced garlic. Sauté until the onion is transparent and aromatic.

Add Broccoli and Spinach:

- Add the cooked broccoli florets and fresh spinach leaves to the saucepan. Sauté for a few more minutes until the spinach wilts.

Blend Ingredients:

- Transfer the sautéed veggies to your Vitamix blender. Add vegetable broth and almond milk.

Blend Until Smooth:

- Start mixing on low speed and gradually raise to high. Blend until the mixture is smooth and creamy.

Adjust Consistency:

- Add extra vegetable broth or almond milk to obtain your preferred consistency if the soup is too thick.

Season and Taste:

- Return the blended soup to the pot and heat it moderately—season with salt and black pepper to taste. Stir thoroughly.

Serve and Enjoy:

- Spoon the Creamy Broccoli and Spinach Soup into dishes. Garnish with optional toppings like grated

Parmesan, croutons, or a drizzle of olive oil. Enjoy the soothing tastes and nourishing deliciousness!

This Creamy Broccoli and Spinach Soup blends the freshness of green veggies with the richness of almond milk for a creamy and nutrient-packed dinner. Adjust the spice and add your favourite toppings to improve the flavour. It's a great way to enjoy a friendly and wholesome soup.

Quinoa and Black Bean Burgers

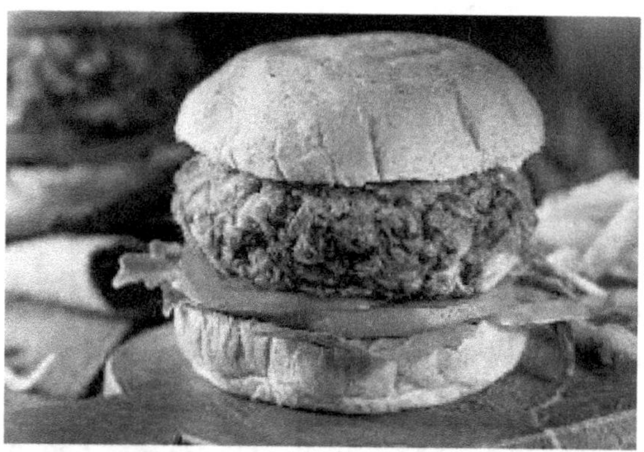

Savour the deliciousness of plant-based protein with these Quinoa and Black Bean Burgers. Packed with nutritional ingredients, these burgers are a tasty and fulfilling alternative to typical meat-based patties.

Ingredients:

- 1 cup cooked quinoa
- One can (15 oz) black beans, drained and rinsed
- ½ cup breadcrumbs (whole wheat or gluten-free)
- ¼ cup coarsely chopped red onion

- Two cloves garlic, minced
- One teaspoon of ground cumin
- One teaspoon of chilli powder
- ½ teaspoon smoked paprika
- Salt and black pepper to taste
- Olive oil for cooking
- Whole wheat burger buns or lettuce wraps
- **Toppings:** lettuce, tomato slices, avocado, onion, etc.

Instructions:

Prepare the Mixture:

- Mash the black beans with a fork until nearly smooth in a mixing basin. Add cooked quinoa, breadcrumbs, finely diced red onion, minced garlic, ground cumin, chilli powder, smoked paprika, salt, and black pepper. Mix thoroughly until all components are incorporated.

Form Patties:

- Divide the ingredients into equal pieces and form them into burger patties. The size might change dependent on your taste.

Cook the Burgers:

- Heat a skillet over medium heat and add a drizzle of olive oil. Place the patties in the skillet and cook for approximately 4-5 minutes on each side until golden brown and cooked through.

- Toast the whole wheat burger buns if desired. Place a burger patty on the bottom bread. Top with your favourite toppings like lettuce, tomato slices, avocado, and onion. Place the top bun on the constructed burger.

- Serve the Quinoa and Black Bean Burgers with a serving of sweet potato fries, a salad, or your favourite side dish. Enjoy plant-based deliciousness and delightful tastes!

These Quinoa and Black Bean Burgers are a tasty and healthful choice for a vegetarian lunch. Customize the spices
Add toppings to suit your taste preferences. They're great for a healthful and substantial lunch or supper.

Zucchini Noodles with Avocado Pesto

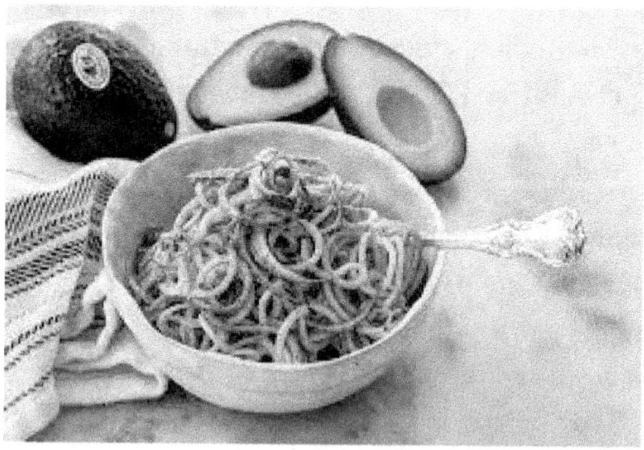

Experience a light, refreshing spin on pasta with Zucchini Noodles with Avocado Pesto. This recipe is tasty and filled with nutritional components, making it a fantastic option for a wholesome supper.

For the Avocado Pesto:

- One ripe avocado, pitted and peeled
- 1 cup fresh basil leaves
- ¼ cup pine nuts or walnuts
- Two cloves garlic
- Juice of 1 lemon
- ¼ cup extra-virgin olive oil
- Salt and black pepper to taste
- **Optional:** grated Parmesan cheese

For the Zucchini Noodles:

- Four medium zucchinis spiralized into noodles
- Olive oil for sautéing
- Salt and black pepper to taste
- Optional toppings: cherry tomatoes, red pepper flakes, additional basil

Instructions:

Prepare Avocado Pesto:

- Add the ripe avocado, fresh basil leaves, pine nuts (or walnuts), garlic, lemon juice, and extra-virgin olive oil in your Vitamix blender. Blend until smooth.

- Add salt, black pepper, and grated Parmesan cheese (if wanted) to the avocado mixture. Blend again to combine the flavours.

- Heat a skillet over medium heat and add a drizzle of olive oil. Sauté the spiralized zucchini noodles for 2-3 minutes until slightly softened—season with salt and black pepper.

- Toss the sautéed zucchini noodles with the avocado pesto until fully covered.

- Top the zucchini noodles with half cherry tomatoes, red pepper flakes for a bite, and additional basil leaves for freshness.

- Serve the Zucchini Noodles with Avocado Pesto as a light and tasty supper. It's a superb alternative to classic spaghetti that's both nutritional and enjoyable.

This Zucchini Noodles with Avocado Pesto meal is a terrific way to experience the smoothness of avocado and the freshness of basil. Customize the toppings and add-ons to build a cuisine that meets your taste preferences. It's a fantastic option for a light lunch or supper.

Spicy Lentil Curry

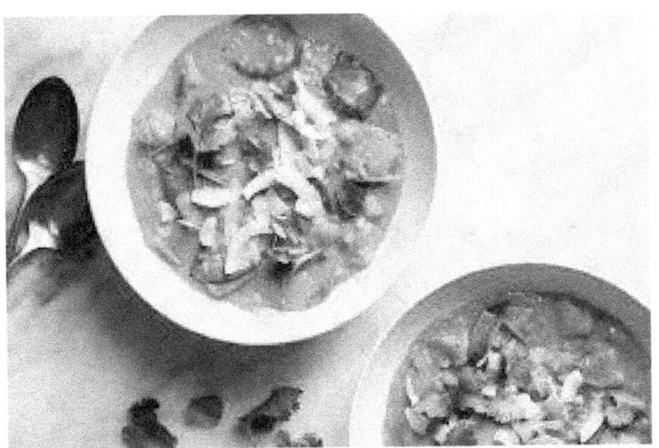

Satisfy your taste buds with the strong flavour of Spicy Lentil Curry. This substantial and healthy recipe is a lovely way to experience the richness of lentils and toasty spices.

Ingredients:

- 1 cup dry green or brown lentils, washed and drained
- 1 onion, finely chopped
- 2 cloves garlic, minced
- One tablespoon of fresh ginger, minced
- One can (14 oz) diced tomatoes
- 1 can (14 oz) coconut milk
- 1 cup vegetable broth one tablespoon curry powder
- 1 teaspoon ground cumin
- ½ teaspoon ground turmeric
- ½ teaspoon chilli powder (adjust to taste)
- ½ teaspoon paprika
- Salt and black pepper to taste

- 2 tablespoons olive oil
- Fresh cilantro for garnish
- Cooked rice or naan bread for serving

Instructions:

Sauté Aromatics:

- Heat olive oil in a saucepan over medium heat. Add chopped onion, minced garlic, and minced ginger. Sauté until the onion is transparent and aromatic.

Add Spices:

- Add curry powder, ground cumin, turmeric, chilli powder, and paprika to the saucepan. Stir and simmer for a minute until the spices are aromatic.

Cook Lentils:

- Add washed lentils, chopped tomatoes (with their juices), coconut milk, and vegetable broth to the saucepan. Stir well to mix.

Simmer Curry:

- Bring the mixture to a boil, then decrease the heat to low. Cover the saucepan and let the curry simmer for approximately 20-25 minutes or until the lentils are cooked.

Adjust Seasoning:

- Taste the curry and adjust the spice by adding salt and black pepper to taste. You may also modify the amount of spiciness by adding extra chilli powder if desired.

Serve:

- Serve the Spicy Lentil Curry over cooked rice or with naan bread. Garnish with fresh cilantro leaves for a blast of colour and flavour.

- Enjoy the rich and comforting flavours of this Spicy Lentil Curry. It's a delicious main meal with protein and excellent for cold days.

This Spicy Lentil Curry is a fantastic way to experience the healthy qualities of lentils coupled with fragrant spices. Feel free to alter the degree of spiciness to your desire. Serve it with your favourite accompaniments for a hearty and savoury supper.

Roasted Red Pepper and Chickpea Hummus Wrap

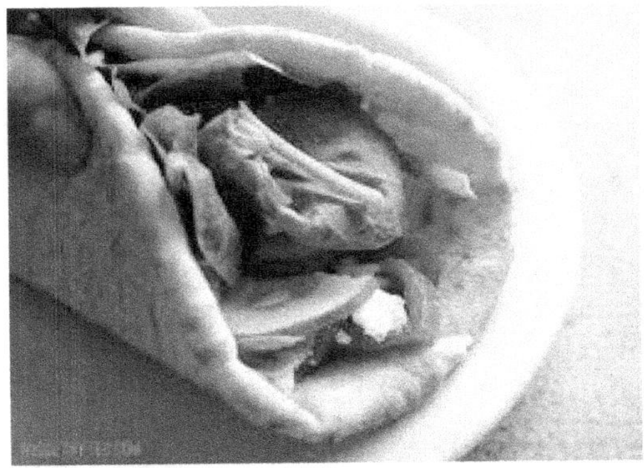

Enjoy savoury and gratifying Roasted Red Pepper and Chickpea Hummus Wrap that's both nutritional and delicious. Packed with plant-based protein and colourful spices, this wrap is excellent for a fast and healthful supper.

- For the Roasted Red Pepper Hummus:
- One can (15 oz) chickpeas, drained and rinsed
- ½ cup roasted red peppers (from a jar or handmade)
- ¼ cup tahini
- Two cloves garlic, minced
- Juice of 1 lemon
- Two tablespoons of olive oil
- ½ teaspoon ground cumin
- Salt and black pepper to taste
- For the Wrap:
- Whole wheat tortilla wraps
- Baby spinach or mixed greens
- Sliced cucumber
- Sliced red onion
- Sliced avocado
- **Optional:** feta cheese or vegan cheese

Instructions:

Prepare Roasted Red Pepper Hummus:

- Add chickpeas, roasted red peppers, tahini, minced garlic, lemon juice, olive oil, ground cumin, salt, and black pepper in your Vitamix blender. Blend until smooth and creamy.

Assemble Wrap:

- Lay a whole wheat tortilla on a clean surface. Spread a liberal dollop of the Roasted Red Pepper Hummus over the tortilla.

- Layer baby spinach or mixed greens, sliced cucumber, sliced red onion, and sliced avocado over the hummus.

- If desired, add crumbled feta or vegan cheese over the veggies for an extra layer of flavour.

- Carefully roll up the wrap, tucking in the sides as you go. Slice the wrap in half diagonally if desired.

- Enjoy the Roasted Red Pepper and Chickpea Hummus Wrap as a healthy lunch or supper. It's a terrific alternative for a portable and tasty dinner on the road.

This Roasted Red Pepper and Chickpea Hummus Wrap is a terrific way to experience the creaminess of hummus and the freshness of veggies. Customize the wrap with your preferred fillings and add-ons to suit your taste preferences. It's a flexible and healthful alternative for a pleasant supper.

Green Goddess Pasta

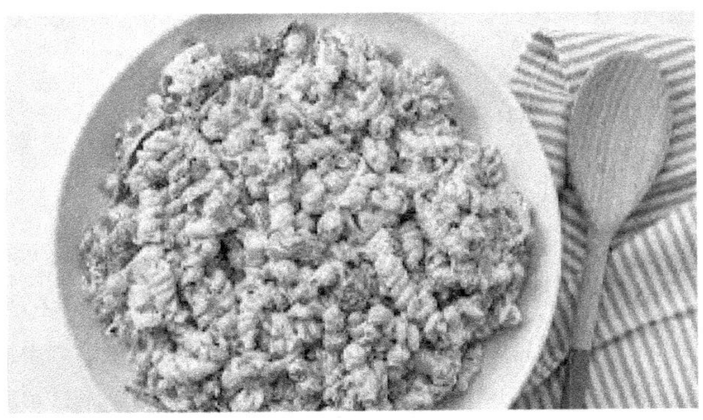

Indulge in the colourful tastes of Green Goddess Pasta, where a creamy green sauce created from fresh ingredients produces a pleasant and healthful meal. This spaghetti is a celebration of greens and herbs that are as tasty as it is nutritious.

Ingredients:

For the Green Sauce:

- 2 cups fresh spinach leaves
- 1 cup fresh basil leaves
- ½ cup fresh parsley leaves
- ¼ cup pine nuts or walnuts
- Two cloves garlic
- Juice of 1 lemon
- ½ cup extra-virgin olive oil
- Salt and black pepper to taste

For the Pasta:

- 12 oz whole wheat or gluten-free pasta
- Olive oil for sautéing
- Sliced cherry tomatoes
- Freshly grated Parmesan cheese or vegan cheese (optional)
- Red pepper flakes for a kick (optional)

Instructions:

Prepare Green Sauce:

- Add fresh spinach, basil, parsley, pine nuts (or walnuts), garlic, lemon juice, and extra-virgin olive oil in your Vitamix blender. Blend until smooth and vivid.

- Add salt and black pepper to the green sauce. Blend again to combine the flavours.

- Cook the pasta according to the package directions until al dente. Drain and put aside.

- In a skillet, heat a drizzle of olive oil over medium heat. Add sliced cherry tomatoes and sauté until they are slightly softened.

- In a large mixing basin, toss the cooked pasta with the green sauce until the pasta is thoroughly covered.

- Gently fold in the sautéed cherry tomatoes, ensuring they are uniformly distributed.

- Divide the Green Goddess Pasta among serving dishes. Add freshly grated Parmesan or vegan cheese over the noodles if preferred. Add a sprinkle of red pepper flakes for added spice.

- Delight in the fresh and colourful flavours of our Green Goddess Pasta. It's a beautiful recipe that combines the benefits of greens, herbs, and nutritious pasta.

This Green Goddess Pasta gives a fresh and healthful spin on typical pasta recipes. Customize the ingredients and add-ons to create a cuisine that meets your tastes. Enjoy a tasty and healthy lunch that's brimming with the freshness of fresh herbs and veggies.

Mushroom Walnut Bolognese

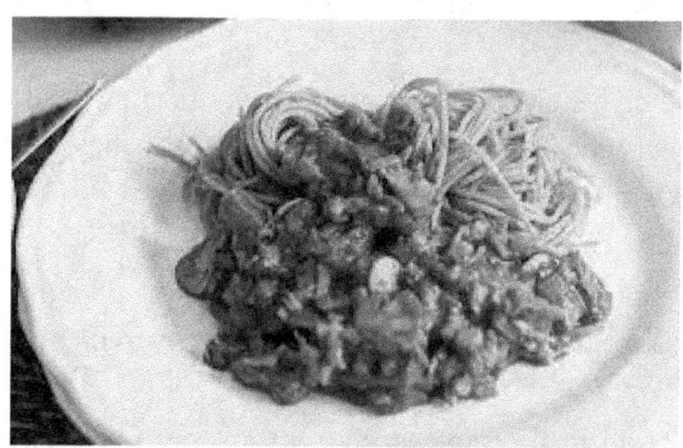

Experience the rich and hearty tastes of a plant-based Mushroom Walnut Bolognese. This recipe is a lovely alternative to classic meat-based bolognese, combining the umami of mushrooms with the crunch of walnuts for a fulfilling lunch.

Ingredients:

- 2 cups cremini mushrooms, coarsely chopped
- 1 cup walnuts, chopped one onion, finely chopped
- Two cloves garlic, minced
- 1 carrot, finely chopped
- One celery stalk, finely chopped
- One can (14 oz) diced tomatoes
- ¼ cup tomato paste

- ½ cup vegetarian broth one teaspoon dried oregano
- One teaspoon of dried basil
- ½ teaspoon dried thyme
- Salt and black pepper to taste
- Olive oil for sautéing
- Cooked whole wheat or gluten-free pasta
- Fresh parsley for garnish
- Vegan or regular grated Parmesan cheese for topping (optional)

Instructions:

Sauté Aromatics:

- In a large skillet, heat olive oil over medium heat. Add chopped onion, minced garlic, diced carrot, and chopped celery. Sauté until the veggies are cooked, and the onion is transparent.

Add Mushrooms and Walnuts:

- Add the finely chopped cremini mushrooms and chopped walnuts to the skillet. Cook, stirring regularly, until the mushrooms lose their liquid and the walnuts are toasted.

Tomato Base:

- Stir in the tomato paste and canned diced tomatoes. Add dried oregano, dry basil, and dried thyme. Mix thoroughly to mix.

Simmer Bolognese:

- Pour in the veggie broth and bring the mixture to a boil. Allow it to simmer for approximately 15-20 minutes or until the flavours merge and the sauce thickens.

- Taste the bolognese and adjust the seasoning with salt and black pepper according to your desire.

- Serve the Mushroom Walnut Bolognese over cooked whole wheat or gluten-free spaghetti. Garnish with freshly chopped parsley.

- Sprinkle vegan or conventional grated Parmesan cheese over the bolognese for extra taste.

- Relish the delicious and nutty flavours of this Mushroom Walnut Bolognese. It's a nutritious and fulfilling meal that gives a fresh spin on a traditional favourite.

This Mushroom Walnut Bolognese delivers a delicious combination of textures and tastes. Feel free to alter the recipe by adding your favourite veggies or changing the seasonings. Serve it over your pasta for a comfortable and tasty supper.

Cauliflower and Chickpea Curry

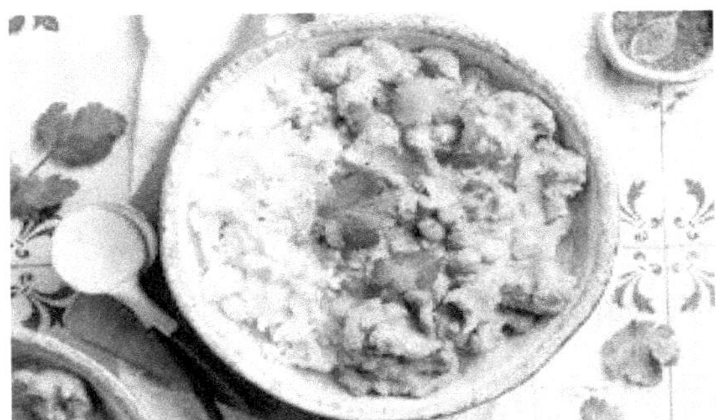

Indulge in the fragrant and savoury delicacy of Cauliflower and Chickpea Curry. This comfortable and healthy recipe mixes cauliflower and chickpeas in a thick, spicy curry sauce that's excellent for a delicious supper.

Ingredients:

- One medium head of cauliflower, chopped into florets
- One can (15 oz) chickpeas, drained and rinsed
- One onion, finely chopped
- Two cloves garlic, minced
- 1 tablespoon fresh ginger, minced
- One can (14 oz) chopped tomatoes
- One can (14 oz) coconut milk
- 1 cup vegetable broth one tablespoon curry powder
- One teaspoon of ground cumin
- ½ teaspoon ground turmeric 1/2 teaspoon ground coriander
- ¼ teaspoon cayenne pepper (adjust to taste)
- Salt and black pepper to taste

- Olive oil for sautéing
- Fresh cilantro for garnish
- Cooked brown rice or naan bread for serving

Instructions:

Sauté Aromatics:

- In a big saucepan or skillet, heat olive oil over medium heat. Add chopped onion, minced garlic, and minced ginger. Sauté until the onion is transparent and aromatic.

Add Spices:

- Add curry powder, ground cumin, turmeric, coriander, and cayenne pepper to the saucepan. Stir and simmer for a minute until the spices are aromatic.

Cook Cauliflower with Chickpeas:

- Add cauliflower florets and drained chickpeas to the saucepan. Stir to coat them with the seasonings.

Tomato and Coconut Base:

- Stir in chopped tomatoes (with their liquids), coconut milk, and vegetable broth.
- Mix thoroughly to mix.

Simmer Curry:

- Bring the mixture to a simmer. Cover the saucepan and let the curry simmer for approximately 20-25 minutes or until the cauliflower is cooked.

Adjust Seasoning:

- Taste the curry and adjust the seasoning with salt and black pepper according to your desire.

- Serve the Cauliflower and Chickpea Curry over cooked brown rice or with naan bread. Garnish with fresh cilantro leaves.

- Enjoy the comforting and fragrant aromas of this Cauliflower and Chickpea Curry. It's a substantial and fulfilling recipe for a warming supper.

This Cauliflower and Chickpea Curry is a lovely way to enjoy the combination of cauliflower and chickpeas in a thick and fragrant sauce. Customize the degree of spiciness and alter the spice to suit your taste. Serve it with your favourite side dishes for a complete and healthful supper.

Savoury Sweet Potato and Black Bean Soup

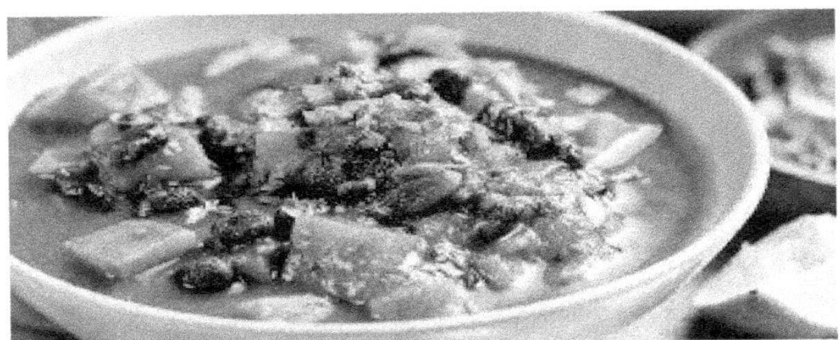

Indulge in the warm and nutritious tastes of Savory Sweet Potato and Black Bean Soup. This substantial soup mixes the sweetness of sweet potatoes with the richness of black beans for a complete and savoury supper.

- Two big sweet potatoes, peeled and chopped
- One can (15 oz) black beans, drained and rinsed
- One onion, chopped
- Two cloves garlic, minced
- One teaspoon of ground cumin
- ½ teaspoon smoked paprika
- ¼ teaspoon ground cinnamon
- Pinch of cayenne pepper (adjust to taste)
- 4 cups vegetable broth
- 1 cup water
- Two tablespoons of olive oil
- Salt and black pepper to taste
- Optional toppings: chopped fresh cilantro, Greek yogurt or coconut yogurt, lime wedges

Instructions:

Sauté Aromatics:

- In a big saucepan, heat olive oil over medium heat. Add chopped onion and minced garlic. Sauté until the onion is transparent and aromatic.

Add Spices:

- Add ground cumin, smoked paprika, ground cinnamon, and a pinch of cayenne pepper to the saucepan. Stir and simmer for a minute until the spices are aromatic.

Cook Sweet Potatoes:

- Add diced sweet potatoes to the saucepan. Stir to coat them with the spices and aromatics.

Add Beans and Broth:

- Pour in the veggie broth and water.
- Add the drained black beans as well. Stir to mix.

Simmer Soup:

- Bring the soup to a simmer. Cover the saucepan and let it boil for approximately 20-25 minutes, or until the sweet potatoes are cooked.

Blend (Optional):

- Use an immersion blender to mix the soup to your chosen consistency, if desired partly. Alternatively, transfer a part of the soup to a blender, process it until smooth, and then return it to the pot.

Season and Serve:

- Taste the soup and adjust the seasoning with salt and black pepper according to your desire.

Serve:

- Ladle the Savory Sweet Potato and Black Bean Soup into bowls. Garnish with chopped fresh cilantro and a dollop of Greek yogurt or coconut yogurt if preferred. Serve with lime wedges for an added punch of flavour.

Enjoy:

- Savour the soothing and hearty flavours of this Savory Sweet Potato and Black Bean Soup. It's a fantastic option for a comfortable and satisfying lunch.

This salty Sweet Potato and Black Bean Soup is a lovely blend of sweet and salty and full of nutrients. Customize the spices and ingredients to make a soup that meets your preferences. Enjoy it as a substantial main meal or a warming side.

Spinach and Feta Stuffed Chicken Breast

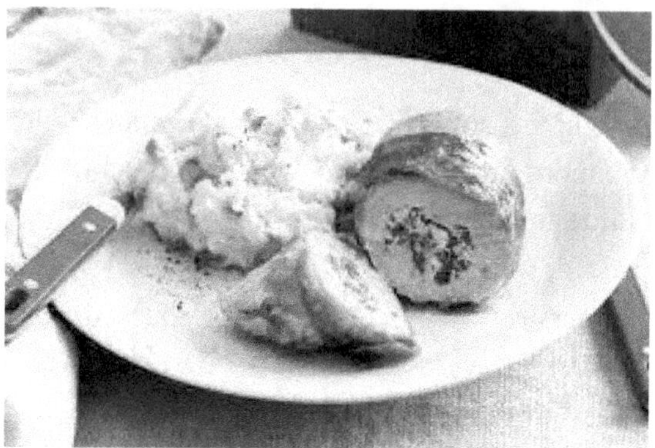

Indulge in a tasty, protein-packed dinner with Spinach and Feta Stuffed Chicken Breast. This dish mixes delicate chicken breast with flavorful stuffing for a delightful and fulfilling supper.

Ingredients:

- Two boneless, skinless chicken breasts
- 1 cup fresh spinach leaves, chopped
- ½ cup crumbled feta cheese
- Two cloves garlic, minced
- One tablespoon of olive oil
- Salt and black pepper to taste
- Toothpicks or kitchen twine
- **Optional:** lemon wedges for serving

Prepare the Filling:

- In a pan, heat olive oil over medium heat. Add minced garlic and chopped spinach. Sauté until the spinach is wilted.
- Remove from heat and mix in crumbled feta cheese. Let the filling cool somewhat.

Preheat the Oven:

- Preheat the oven to 375°F (190°C).

Prepare the Chicken Breasts:

- Use a sharp knife to make a horizontal incision down the side of each chicken breast, forming a pocket without cutting all the way through.

Stuff the Chicken Breasts:

- Divide the spinach and feta mixture between the chicken breasts, carefully tucking it into the pockets.

Secure the Chicken:

- Use toothpicks or kitchen thread to seal the holes in the chicken breasts and prevent the contents from spilling out.

Season the Chicken:

- Season the exterior of the chicken breasts with salt and black pepper.

Sear the Chicken:

- In an oven-safe skillet, heat a little olive oil over medium-high heat. Sear the chicken breasts for approximately 2-3 minutes on each side until golden brown.

Bake the Chicken:

- Transfer the pan to the preheated oven and bake for approximately 15-20 minutes, or until the chicken is cooked through (reaches an internal temperature of 165°F or 74°C).

Rest and Serve:

- Remove the toothpicks or twine before serving. Let the chicken rest for a few minutes before slicing.

Serve:

- Serve the Spinach and Feta Stuffed Chicken Breast with your favourite side dishes. Squeeze fresh lemon juice over the chicken before serving, if preferred.

Enjoy:

- Enjoy this tasty and comforting dinner rich with the benefits of spinach and feta.

This Spinach and Feta Stuffed Chicken Breast is a superb way to elevate chicken into a rich and beautiful supper. Customize the filling and seasoning to suit your taste preferences. Serve it with a choice of sides for a well-balanced and tasty dinner.

CHAPTER EIGHT

Decadent Desserts

Chocolate Avocado Mousse

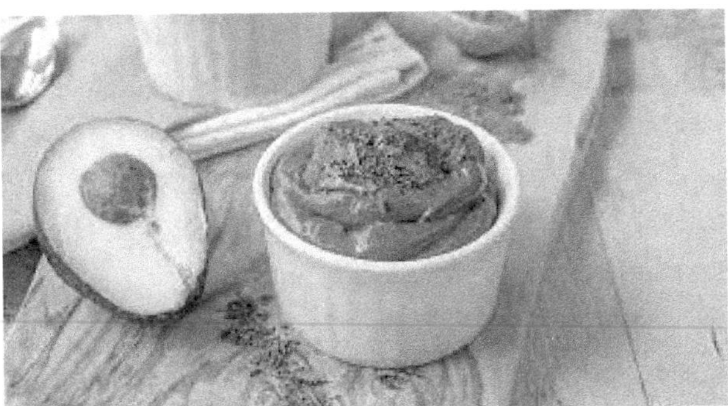

Indulge in the velvety richness of Chocolate Avocado Mousse, a delectable dessert that mixes the creaminess of ripe avocados with the extravagance of chocolate. This delicacy is not only tasty but also healthier than standard mousse recipes.

Ingredients:

- Two ripe avocados peeled and pitted
- ¼ cup cocoa powder
- ¼ cup pure maple syrup or honey
- One teaspoon of vanilla extract and a Pinch of salt
- Optional toppings: whipped coconut cream, berries, chopped almonds, shaved chocolate

Instructions:

Blend the Mousse:

- Add the ripe avocados, chocolate powder, pure maple syrup or honey, vanilla essence, and a sprinkling of salt in your Vitamix blender.

Blend Until Smooth:

- Start mixing on low speed and gradually raise to high. Blend until the mixture is smooth and creamy, scraping down the edges of the blender as required.

Taste and Adjust:

- Taste the mousse and adjust the sweetness by adding extra maple syrup or honey if required.

Chill:

- Transfer the chocolate avocado mousse to serving plates or glasses. Cover and refrigerate for at least 1-2 hours to let the flavours mingle and the mousse cool.

Serve and Garnish:

- Before serving, you may top the mousse with whipped coconut cream, fresh berries, chopped almonds, or shaved chocolate for added texture and taste.

Enjoy:

- Savour the decadent and guilt-free delight of this Chocolate Avocado Mousse. It's a fantastic treat for chocolate fans seeking a healthy dessert choice.

This Chocolate Avocado Mousse is a terrific way to savour the smoothness of avocados while meeting your chocolate cravings. Feel free to alter the sweetness and toppings according to your taste preferences. Serve it as a solitary dessert or as a final touch to a special dinner.

Triple Berry Sorbet

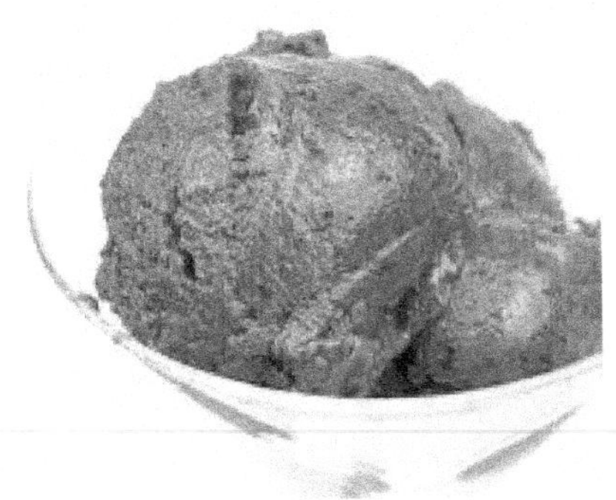

Experience the vivid and refreshing tastes of summer with Triple Berry Sorbet. This delectable delicacy mixes the sweetness of strawberries, blueberries, and raspberries into a naturally flavorful and pleasant dessert.

Ingredients:

- 2 cups mixed berries (strawberries, blueberries, raspberries), fresh or frozen
- ¼ cup pure maple syrup or honey
- One tablespoon of freshly squeezed lemon juice
- ½ cup water (modify as required)
- Optional: fresh mint leaves for garnish

Instructions:

Prepare the Berries:

- If using fresh berries, rinse and remove any stems or leaves. If using frozen berries, you may defrost them somewhat.

Blend the Sorbet:

- Add mixed berries, pure maple syrup or honey, freshly squeezed lemon juice, and water in your Vitamix blender.

Blend Until Smooth:

- Start mixing on low speed and gradually raise to high. Blend until the mixture is smooth and the berries are entirely integrated.

Taste and Adjust:

- Taste the sorbet base and adjust the sweetness by adding extra maple syrup or honey if required. You may also tweak the tartness with a touch of extra lemon juice.

Chill the Mixture:

- Transfer the sorbet mixture to a container and cover it. Place it in the refrigerator to cool for approximately 1-2 hours.

Freeze the Sorbet:

- Once the mixture is cold, pour it into an ice cream machine and churn according to the manufacturer's directions.
- If you don't have an ice cream machine, pour the mixture into a shallow container and set it in the freezer.

- Every 30 minutes, stir the mixture with a fork to break up ice crystals until it achieves the desired sorbet consistency.

- Scoop the Triple Berry Sorbet into serving dishes or glasses.
- Garnish with fresh mint leaves for a blast of colour and scent.

- Delight in the refreshing and delicious aromas of our Triple Berry Sorbet. It's a fantastic way to chill down and savour the flavour of ripe berries.

This Triple Berry Sorbet is a terrific way to appreciate the wealth of summer berries. Customize the sweetness and balance of tastes to your preference. Serve it as a light, refreshing dessert or a palette cleanser between meals.

Salted Caramel Date Shake

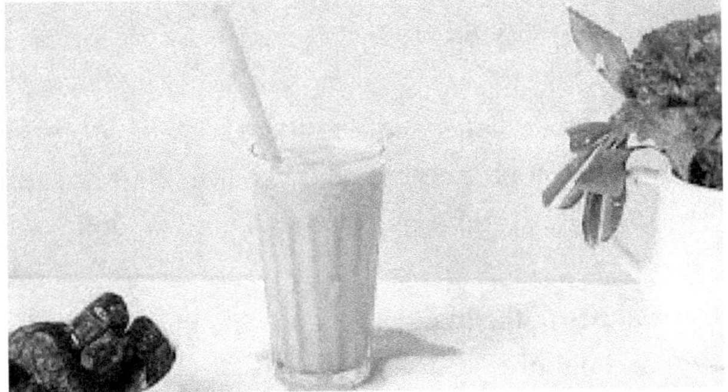

Satisfy your sweet craving with the rich and delicious flavours of a Salted Caramel Date Shake. This delectable dessert mixes the natural sweetness of dates with the richness of caramel and a tinge of saltiness.

- 6-8 Medjool dates, pitted and soaked in warm water for 10 minutes
- 1 cup almond milk or any milk of your choosing
- ¼ teaspoon vanilla extract
- Pinch of salt
- One tablespoon of pure maple syrup (optional for extra sweetness)
- Ice cubes
- Whipped coconut cream (for topping)
- Caramel sauce (for drizzling, optional)
- Flakey sea salt (for garnish)

Instructions:

Soak Dates:

- Pit the Medjool dates in warm water for approximately 10 minutes to soften them.

Blend the Shake:

- Drain the soaked dates and add them to your Vitamix mixer. Add almond milk, vanilla essence, a bit of salt, and pure maple syrup if using. Blend until smooth.

Add Ice:

- Add ice cubes to the blender and process until the drink is cool and bubbly.

- Taste the shake and adjust the sweetness and saltiness according to your desire. You may add extra maple syrup or salt as required.

- Pour the Salted Caramel Date Shake into glasses.

- Top the shake with a dollop of whipped coconut cream. Drizzle caramel sauce over the top for an added touch of indulgence.

- Sprinkle a teaspoon of flakey sea salt over the whipped cream for that right blend of sweet and salty.

- Savour the rich and delightful tastes of our Salted Caramel Date Shake. It's a fantastic way to savour the sweetness of dates in a pleasant and decadent dessert.

This Salted Caramel Date Shake is a fantastic alternative for seeking something sweet and decadent. Customize the sweetness and saltiness to suit your taste preferences, and enjoy this delight as a dessert or a special indulgence.

Peanut Butter Chocolate Protein Shake

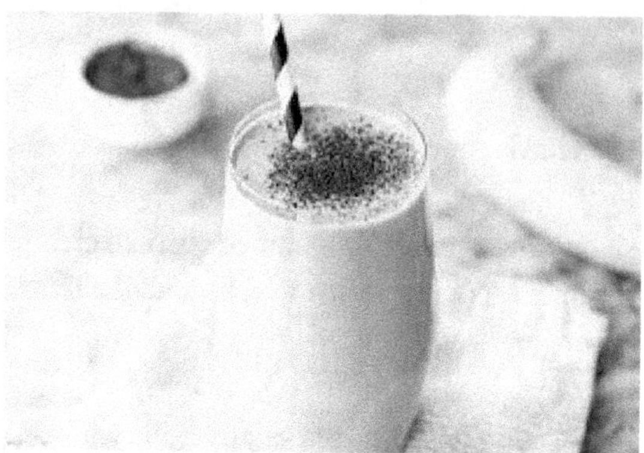

Indulge in the iconic peanut butter and chocolate combo while upping your protein consumption with this delightful Peanut Butter Chocolate Protein Shake. This smoothie is delicious and filling and a terrific alternative for a post-workout recovery or a fast and healthy snack.

Ingredients:

- One scoop of chocolate protein powder
- Two teaspoons of natural peanut butter
- 1 tablespoon cocoa powder
- 1 ripe banana
- 1 cup almond milk or any milk of your choosing
- ½ cup ice cubes
- Optional: Honey or maple syrup for extra sweetness
- **Optional toppings:** crushed peanuts, chocolate chips, banana slices

Instructions:

Prepare Ingredients:

- Peel and slice the ripe banana.

Blend the Shake:

- Add the chocolate protein powder, natural peanut butter, cocoa powder, sliced banana, almond milk, and ice cubes in your Vitamix blender.

Blend Until Smooth:

- Start mixing on low speed and gradually raise to high. Blend until all the ingredients are fully incorporated, and the smoothie is smooth and creamy.

Taste and Adjust:

- Taste the shake and add honey or maple syrup if you want it sweeter.

Serve:

- Pour the Peanut Butter Chocolate Protein Shake into a glass.

Top and Garnish:

- Top the shake with crushed peanuts, chocolate chips, or banana slices for extra texture and taste.

Enjoy:

- Enjoy the pleasant and healthful tastes of our Peanut Butter Chocolate Protein Shake. It's a beautiful option for a fast and tasty protein-packed treat.

This Peanut Butter Chocolate Protein Shake is an excellent way to replenish after a workout or to enjoy as a tasty snack. Customize the sweetness and texture to your preference, and feel free to add your favourite protein powder for an additional protein boost.

Mango Coconut Ice Cream

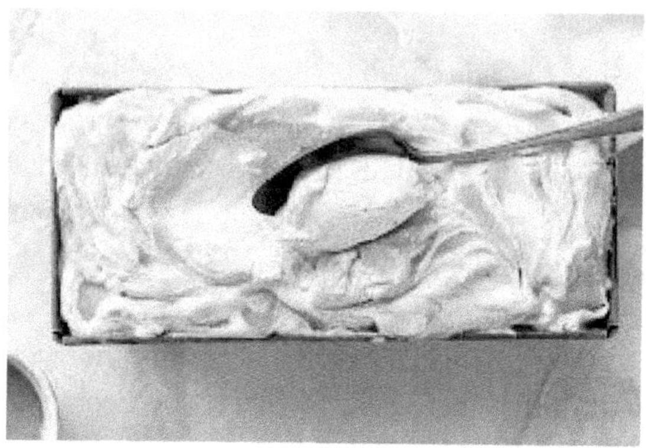

Experience the tropical ecstasy of Mango Coconut Ice Cream, a creamy and delightful delicacy that mixes the sweetness of mangoes with the richness of coconut milk. This dairy-free dessert is a fantastic way to savour the tastes of summer.

Ingredients:

- 2 cups ripe mango chunks (fresh or frozen)
- One can (14 oz) full-fat coconut milk
- ¼ cup pure maple syrup or honey
- One teaspoon of vanilla extract
- Pinch of salt
- Optional: crushed coconut for additional texture
- Optional toppings: fresh mango chunks, mint leaves

Instructions:

Prepare Mango Chunks:

- If using fresh mango, peel and slice the mango into pieces. If using frozen mango, make sure it's somewhat thawed.

Blend the Ice Cream Base:

- Add the ripe mango chunks, full-fat coconut milk, pure maple syrup or honey, vanilla essence, and a touch of salt in your Vitamix blender.

Blend Until Smooth:

- Start mixing on low speed and gradually raise to high. Blend until the mixture is smooth and creamy.

Taste and Adjust:

- Taste the ice cream base and adjust the sweetness by adding extra maple syrup or honey if required.

Chill the Mixture:

- Transfer the ice cream mixture to a container and cover it. Place it in the refrigerator to cool for approximately 1-2 hours.

Churn the Ice Cream:

- Pour the cold mixture into an ice cream maker and churn according to the manufacturer's directions. If you don't have an ice cream machine, pour the mixture into a shallow container and set it in the freezer. Every 30 minutes, stir the liquid with a fork to break up ice crystals until it achieves the desired ice cream consistency.

- Scoop the Mango Coconut Ice Cream into dishes. Garnish with fresh mango slices, shredded coconut, or mint leaves for an added touch of tropical flare.

- Delight in the creamy and refreshing tastes of our Mango Coconut Ice Cream. It's a fantastic way to savour the sweetness of mangoes and the creaminess of coconut.

This Mango Coconut Ice Cream is a terrific way to capture the spirit of summer in a delectable treat. Customize the sweetness and toppings to your liking, and enjoy it as a refreshing treat on a warm day or as a special indulgence anytime.

Frozen Mixed Berry Cheesecake Bites

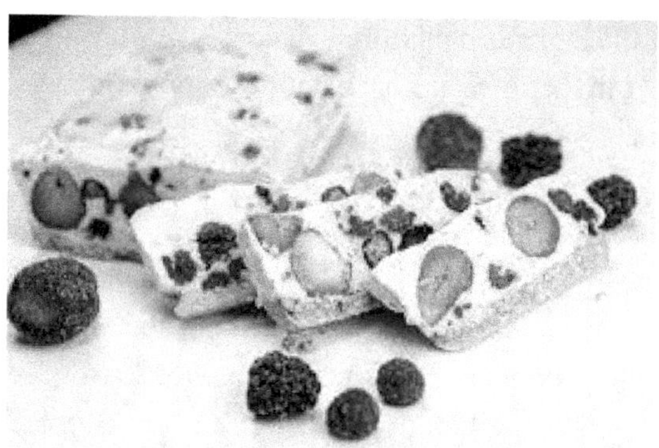

Indulge in the deliciousness of Frozen Mixed Berry Cheesecake Bites, a wonderful delicacy that mixes the creamy richness of cheesecake with the vivid tastes of mixed berries.

These bite-sized sweets are excellent for a sweet and refreshing delight.

- 1 cup graham cracker crumbs
- Three tablespoons unsalted butter melted two teaspoons granulated sugar For the Cheesecake Filling:
- 8 oz cream cheese, softened
- ½ cup powdered sugar
- One teaspoon of vanilla extract
- ½ cup thick cream

- ½ cup mixed berries (strawberries, blueberries, raspberries)
- Two teaspoons of granulated sugar
- One teaspoon of lemon juice

- **Crush Graham Crackers:** In a food processor or Vitamix blender, grind the graham crackers until they turn into fine crumbs.
- **Combine Crumbs and Butter:** In a bowl, combine the graham cracker crumbs, melted butter, and granulated sugar. Mix until the mixture resembles wet sand.

- **Line tin:** Line a miniature muffin tin with paper liners.
- **Add Crust:** Divide the crust mixture equally among the muffin cups. Press the ingredients down with the back of a spoon to produce a tight crust.

Prepare the Cheesecake Filling:

- **Whip Cream Cheese:** Wash the softened cream cheese in a mixing basin until smooth.
- **Add Sugar and Vanilla:** Add the powdered sugar and vanilla essence to the cream cheese. Mix until thoroughly blended and smooth.
- **Beat Cream:** In a separate dish, beat the heavy cream until firm peaks form.
- **Fold Cream into Cream Cheese Mixture:** Gently fold the whipped cream into the cream cheese mixture until thoroughly mixed. This provides a light and creamy cheesecake filling.

Prepare the Berry Swirl:

- **Combine Berries:** In your Vitamix blender, combine the mixed berries, granulated sugar, and lemon juice until smooth. Strain the mixture to remove any seeds if desired.

Assemble and Freeze:

- **Layer Cheesecake and Berry Swirl:** Spoon a cheesecake filling over the crust in each muffin cup. Add a tiny dollop of the berry swirl on the cheesecake layer.
- **Produce Swirls:** Use a toothpick or a tiny stick to gently swirl the berry mixture into the cheesecake mixture to produce a marbled look.

- **Freeze:** Place the muffin pan in the freezer and freeze until the cheesecake bits are tricky, generally for approximately 4-6 hours or overnight.

- **Serve and Enjoy:** Remove the cheesecake bits from the muffin tray once frozen. Let them rest at room temperature for a few minutes before serving. Enjoy these delectable Frozen Mixed Berry Cheesecake Bites as a beautiful and refreshing treat.

These Frozen Mixed Berry Cheesecake Bites deliver the right blend of creamy cheesecake and delicious berry swirls. Customize the fruit mix and enjoy these bite-sized sweets as a refreshing dessert on a warm day or an elegant addition to any party.

Chocolate Banana Nice Cream

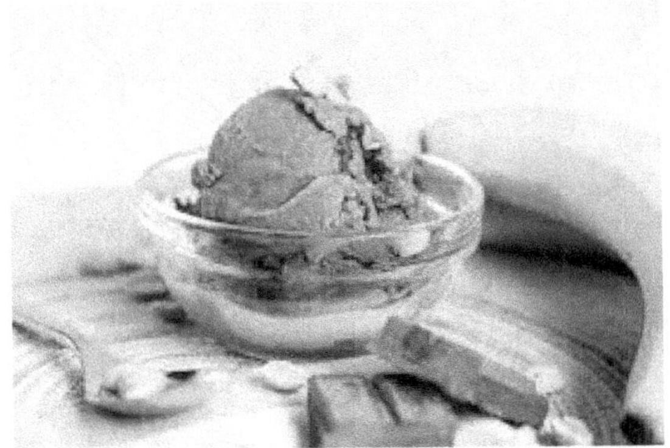

Indulge in the creamy and delicious tastes of Chocolate Banana Nice Cream, a delectable frozen dessert from only two essential ingredients: ripe bananas and chocolate powder. This healthier alternative to regular ice cream will fulfill your chocolate cravings.

Ingredients:

- 3-4 ripe bananas, peeled, sliced, and frozen
- Two teaspoons of unsweetened cocoa powder
- Optional: a dash of almond milk or any milk of your choosing
- Optional toppings: chopped almonds, chocolate chips, sliced bananas

Instructions:

Prepare and Freeze Bananas:

- Peel the ripe bananas, slice them into coins, and set the banana slices in a single layer on a parchment-lined plate. Freeze until they are firm, generally for a few hours or overnight.

Blend the Nice Cream:

- Place the frozen banana slices in your Vitamix blender. Add the unsweetened cocoa powder.

Blend Until Creamy:

- Start mixing on low speed and gradually raise to high. If the mixture has problems mixing, you may add a little splash of almond milk or your chosen milk to assist it. Blend until the mixture is creamy and smooth.

Taste and Adjust:

- If preferred, taste the excellent cream and modify the sweetness by adding a drizzle of honey or maple syrup.

The natural sweetness of the ripe bananas should be plenty for most tastes.

- Scoop the Chocolate Banana Nice Cream into bowls.

- If desired, sprinkle chopped nuts, chocolate chips, or sliced bananas on top for extra texture and taste.

- Savour the rich and delightful tastes of our Chocolate Banana Nice Cream. It's a fantastic way to savour the smoothness of bananas and the pleasure of chocolate.

This Chocolate Banana Nice Cream is a guilt-free dessert alternative that's easy to create and wonderfully tasty. Customize the toppings and sweetness to suit your taste preferences, and enjoy it as a delightful treat anytime your sweet craving calls.

Almond Butter Brownies

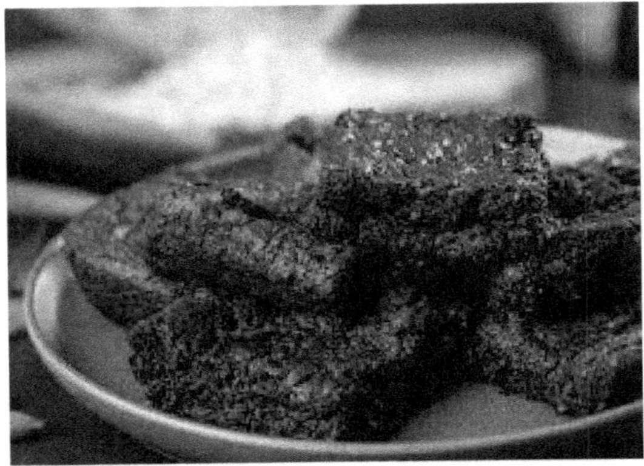

Indulge in the rich and nutty tastes of Almond Butter Brownies, a delicious take on the traditional chocolate delicacy. These brownies are baked with almond butter for a nutty and delicious flavour guaranteed to fulfill your sweet desires.

Ingredients:

For the Brownies:

- ½ cup almond butter (creamy or crunchy)
- ¼ cup melted coconut oil
- ½ cup cocoa powder
- ½ cup coconut sugar or granulated sugar
- Two big eggs
- One teaspoon of vanilla extract
- ¼ teaspoon salt
- ¼ teaspoon baking powder
- Optional Additions:
- ½ cup chocolate chips
- Chopped almonds for topping

Instructions:

Preheat the Oven:

- Preheat your oven to 350°F (175°C). Grease or line an 8x8-inch baking tray with parchment paper.

Mix Wet Ingredients:

- Whisk together the almond butter, melted coconut oil, and coconut sugar in a mixing bowl until thoroughly blended and smooth.

Add Eggs and Vanilla:

- Add the eggs and vanilla essence to the almond butter mixture. Whisk until the mixture is thoroughly mixed.

Incorporate Dry Ingredients:

- Add the cocoa powder, salt, and baking powder to the wet ingredients. Mix until everything is well combined.

Optional Chocolate Chips:

- If desired, mix in the chocolate chips to give more chocolaty pleasure to the brownie batter.

Pour into Pan:

- Pour the brownie batter into the prepared baking pan. Use a spatula to distribute it evenly.

Bake the Brownies:

- Bake in the preheated oven for approximately 20-25 minutes or until a toothpick inserted into the middle comes out with a few wet crumbs. Be cautious not to overbake since almond butter brownies may dry out if cooked too long.

Cool and Slice:

- Allow the brownies to cool in the pan briefly before transferring to a wire rack to cool fully. Once chilled, slice into squares.

Serve and Enjoy:

- Enjoy these Almond Butter Brownies as a lovely and nutty variation on classic brownies. You may also top them with chopped almonds for extra texture and nuttiness.

These Almond Butter Brownies are a fantastic treat for individuals who appreciate the rich taste of almond butter. They're a superb alternative for a memorable dessert or a lovely snack. Customize the recipe by adding your favourite mix-ins or toppings for a distinctive touch.

Strawberry Cashew Cream Tart

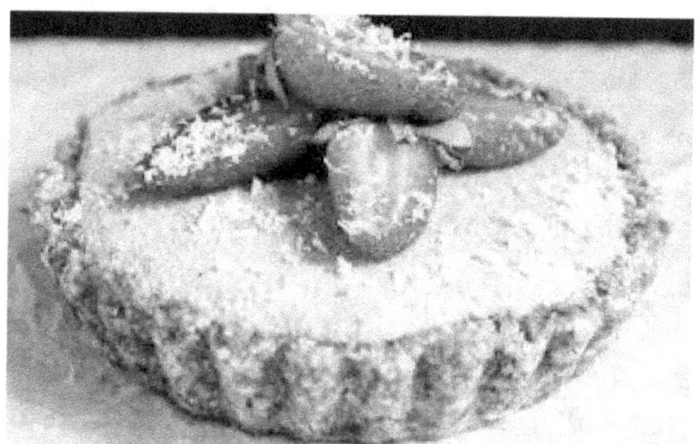

Indulge in the creamy and delicious tastes of Strawberry Cashew Cream Tart, a delectable dessert with a nutty cashew cream filling and a bright strawberry topping. This tart is not only tasty but also dairy-free and vegan.

Ingredients:

For the Crust:

- 1 cup almond flour
- ¼ cup coconut flour
- Two teaspoons of melted coconut oil
- Two tablespoons of pure maple syrup or honey

Pinch of salt For the Cashew Cream Filling:

- 1 ½ cups raw cashews, soaked for at least 4 hours or overnight, then drained
- ¼ cup coconut cream
- ¼ cup pure maple syrup or honey
- ¼ cup melted coconut oil
- One teaspoon of vanilla extract

Pinch of salt For the Strawberry Topping:

- 2 cups fresh strawberries, hulled and sliced
- One tablespoon of pure maple syrup or honey

Instructions:

Preheat the Oven:

- Preheat your oven to 350°F (175°C).

Mix the Crust:

- Add almond flour, coconut flour, melted coconut oil, pure maple syrup or honey, and a sprinkle of salt in a mixing bowl. Mix until the ingredients come together and form a dough.

Press into Tart Pan:

- Press the dough into a tart pan, evenly covering the bottom and sides. Use your fingers or the back of a spoon to create a uniform coating.

Bake the Crust:

- Bake the crust in the oven for approximately 10-12 minutes or until golden brown. Remove from the oven and allow it to cool fully.

Prepare the Cashew Cream Filling:

- **Blend the Cashew Cream:** In your Vitamix blender, add the soaked and drained cashews, coconut cream, pure maple syrup or honey, melted coconut oil, vanilla extract, and a touch of salt. Blend until the mixture is smooth and creamy.

Assemble the Tart:

Spread the Cashew Cream:

- Spread the cashew cream filling over the chilled tart shell, making an equal layer.
- Arrange Strawberry Topping:
- Mix the cut strawberries with pure maple syrup or honey in a dish. Arrange the strawberry slices on top of the cashew cream filling.

Chill:

- Place the tart in the refrigerator for at least 1-2 hours, allowing the flavours to mingle and the filling to the firm.

Serve and Enjoy:

- Slice and serve the Strawberry Cashew Cream Tart as a beautiful and refreshing dessert. The mix of creamy cashew filling and juicy strawberries is a delicious treat.

This Strawberry Cashew Cream Tart is an excellent alternative for people wanting a dairy-free and vegan treat. Customize the sweetness and toppings of your choice, and enjoy this exquisite dessert as a perfect finale for dinner or a special occasion.

Coconut Chocolate Pudding

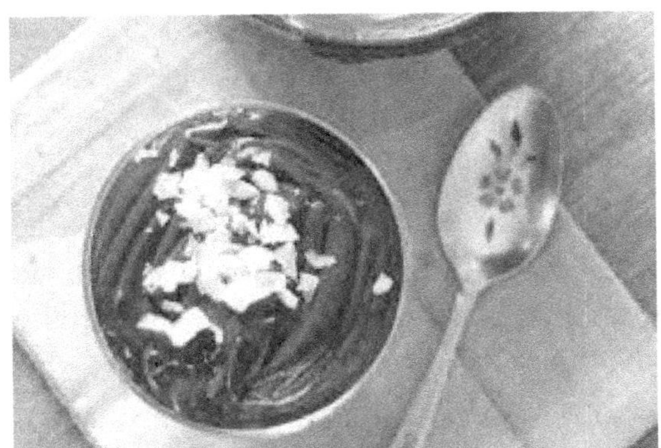

Indulge in the creamy and chocolaty bliss of Coconut Chocolate Pudding, a delectable dessert that mixes the richness of chocolate with the tropical taste of coconut. This dairy-free and vegan pudding is guaranteed to fulfill your sweet desires.

Ingredients:

- One can (14 oz) full-fat coconut milk
- ¼ cup cocoa powder
- ¼ cup pure maple syrup or honey
- ¼ teaspoon vanilla extract
- Pinch of salt
- Two tablespoons cornstarch or arrowroot powder
- **Optional toppings:** shaved coconut, chopped nuts, fresh fruit

Instructions:

- **Mix Cornstarch:** In a small bowl, mix the cornstarch or arrowroot powder with a couple of teaspoons of coconut milk to produce a smooth paste. Set aside.

- **Add Ingredients:** In a saucepan, add the remaining coconut milk, cocoa powder, pure maple syrup or honey, vanilla essence, and a sprinkle of salt. Whisk until the mixture is thoroughly blended and smooth.

- **Heat Mixture:** Place the pot over medium heat and bring the mixture to a moderate simmer.

- **Add Cornstarch Paste:** Gradually whisk the cornstarch paste into the boiling liquid. Continue whisking until the pudding starts to thicken, generally for approximately 3-5 minutes.

- **Simmer and Thicken:** Keep the pudding mixture at a low simmer, stirring regularly, until it thickens to a custard-like consistency. This usually takes approximately 5-7 minutes.

- **Take from Heat:** Once the pudding has thickened, remove the pot.

- **Cool and Serve:** Allow the Coconut Chocolate Pudding to cool slightly before transferring it to serving plates or glasses.

- **Cool:** Place the pudding in the refrigerator and set for at least 1-2 hours.

- **Top and Garnish:** Before serving, you may sprinkle shaved coconut, chopped almonds, or fresh berries on top for extra texture and taste.

- **Enjoy:** Savor the creamy and chocolaty deliciousness of our Coconut Chocolate Pudding. It's a fantastic way to experience the tastes of chocolate and coconut in a dairy-free and vegan delight.

This Coconut Chocolate Pudding is a superb dessert choice for individuals who adore chocolate and coconut. Customize the sweetness and toppings to your suit, and enjoy it as a soothing and gratifying dessert after a meal or as a special treat.